The DIABETIC MAN

Other books by June Biermann and Barbara Toohey:

The Peripatetic Diabetic
The Diabetes Question and Answer Book
The Diabetic's Sports & Exercise Book
The Diabetic's Total Health Book
The Diabetic's Book: All Your Questions Answered
The Diabetic Woman (with Lois Jovanovic-Peterson, M.D.)

Other books by Peter A. Lodewick, M.D.:

A Diabetic Doctor Looks at Diabetes: His and Yours

The
DIABETIC
MAN

· · · · ·

A Guide to Health and Success in All Areas of Your Life

With Advice, Empathy, and
Support for Those Who Have a
Diabetic Man in Their Lives

· · · · ·

PETER A. LODEWICK, M.D., and
JUNE BIERMANN and BARBARA TOOHEY

LOWELL HOUSE
Los Angeles
CONTEMPORARY BOOKS
Chicago

Library of Congress Cataloging-in-Publication Data

Lodewick, Peter A.
    The diabetic man: a guide to health and success in all areas of your
life: with advice, empathy, and support for those who have a diabetic man
in their lives/Peter Lodewick, June Biermann, and Barbara Toohey.
        p. cm.
    Includes bibliographical references and index.
    ISBN 0-929923-24-3
    1. Diabetes—Popular works. 2. Men—Diseases. I. Title.
    RC660.4.L64 1991
    616.4'62—dc20   91–4455
                                                                CIP

Requests for such permissions should be addressed to:

Lowell House
1875 Century Park East, Suite 220
Los Angeles, CA 90067

Publisher: Jack Artenstein
Vice-President/Editor-in-Chief: Janice Gallagher
Director of Marketing: Elizabeth Duell Wood
Design: Tanya Maiboroda

Manufactured in the United States of America
10 9 8 7 6 5 4 3 2 1

Contents

Foreword

Women, *The Diabetic Man* is really for us, too! Every wife, girlfriend, roommate, significant other, mother, sister, secretary, aunt, and grandmother of a diabetic man needs to read this book.

Dr. Lodewick has systematically and carefully explained all the reasons why the beloved diabetic man in our lives needs to take such good care of himself. We must support, nurture, and participate in his diabetes management program and above all not undermine or be jealous of his preoccupation. Our efforts will be rewarded as we witness his transformation to a healthy, successful man.

I might as well direct you to the sections that were written for you: The Psychosocial Man, The Sexual Man, and The Diabetic Man in Your Life. In these three chapters, the mysteries of the man in your life are revealed and you learn that as a woman who cares about a diabetic man, you are not alone. You learn that his ups and downs may be related to the swings in his blood sugars. You also learn how hard it is for him to "not be perfect." It is amazing how much easier it is to be sympathetic once you understand the true meaning of mood changes.

Gentlemen, do not worry. Dr. Lodewick has not revealed *all* your secrets, and the book was really written with you in mind. He has covered a wide range of topics, including sports and athletics, work, love, food, traveling, and living with diabetes as a diabetic man. In each instance, he not only explains the facts and the problems but also provides solutions.

As a physician for many diabetic men, I found this book to be a resource not only for my patients but also for me. Dr. Lodewick tells us how to pick the right physician, insisting that the physician be well informed and a good listener. This book has educated me and helped me listen better. Perhaps it could help your physician become a better listener, too.

And, as a woman with diabetes, I picked up tips for myself on exercise, traveling, and health insurance. Quite frankly, the majority of *The Diabetic Man* applies to the Diabetic Woman as well. This book could even be titled *The Diabetic Person*. Thank you, Dr. Lodewick, June, and Barbara for giving us a book for everyone.

Lois Jovanovic-Peterson, M.D.
Coauthor of *The Diabetic Woman*

Introduction

by June Biermann and Barbara Toohey

Several years ago we wrote a book called *The Woman's Holistic Headache Relief Book*. We gave it that title both because it was based on June's experiences with chronic headaches and because more women than men are headache sufferers. Men more often tend to have lower back pain, sometimes called "the male migraine." At any rate, the book told women how to identify the causes of and find the cures for chronic headaches. After it was published, we received many complaints from our readers. The complaints weren't about the contents of the book but about the title. People protested that virtually all the information would be just as applicable and helpful to men as to women, but because of its title, no man would ever pick it up, let alone be caught reading it.

To solve this dilemma, we suggested that another title could be printed on the inside of the dust jacket: *The Man's Macho Headache Relief Book*. Then men could just turn the dust jacket inside out and learn to cure their headaches without shame or embarrassment.

On the other hand, when we wrote *The Diabetic Woman* (with Lois Jovanovic-Peterson, M.D.), absolutely no one suggested that a man could derive as much benefit from it as a woman if he just turned the dust jacket inside out. Although diabetic men and women do have much in common, as participants in co-educational diabetes classes and support groups quickly learn, there are still huge differences between some major problems of diabetic men and those of diabetic women. For example, pregnancy often occupies center stage in a diabetic woman's theater of the mind, while impotency, if not on center stage for men, often seems to be waiting in the wings ready to make its entrance.

3

Also, men and women generally have different attitudes and approaches to health problems. Women, with their pregnancies or monthly periods, are more accustomed to not feeling in prime condition all the time. They are also more willing to make frequent visits to doctors and to work gradually toward improving their health by changing their habits. As traditional nurturers of others, they understand better how to nurture themselves. Many men, in contrast, have little patience with disease. They often adopt an attitude of fix-it-fast-or-forget-it. Since diabetes can't be fixed, men have a far greater tendency to forget their diabetes until they develop constant reminders in the form of complications.

It's significant that when we sent out a message on the diabetes tom-toms via our newsletter, the *Health-O-Gram*, broadcasting the news that we were writing a book on the diabetic woman and asking for questions that women would like to have answered, we were deluged with responses. Many of these questions were almost life stories, pages and pages long, replete with insights, musings, and ponderings on the diabetic condition. When we asked the same of men, we received hardly a reply, and those replies we did receive were terse and to the point. We actually received more questions from women about the diabetic men in their lives than we did from men, and the majority of these questions concerned men who wouldn't take care of themselves.

It was, in fact, women who love diabetic men—their wives, sisters, mothers, lovers, and friends—who first convinced us that this book should be written. In a kind of reverse sexism, we initially felt that men didn't particularly need a book telling them how to fit diabetes into their lives. Compared to the problems diabetic women have to go through, diabetic men have it relatively easy, or so we thought. After all, they can father children without following a rigid program of blood sugar control, without risk to their health and that of their children, and without the heavy additional expenses that diabetic women must pay for the privilege of parenthood. They don't have to put up with the life-long hormonal vagaries that mess up emotions and blood sugars. And they don't have to juggle a multitude of life roles simultaneously as women do. When we think back on it now, our prejudiced attitude was much like that of some Type I (insulin-dependent) diabetics who think that life is a piece of sugar-free cake for Type II's (non-insulin-dependent). But after talking at length with diabetic men and their significant others, we quickly abandoned our reverse sexist attitudes with the realization that men need as much help with their diabetes as women do. They may even need more help because, having had the notions of independence and strength drilled into them since infancy, it's hard for many of them to acknowledge that they need to accept help when it's offered.

When we were convinced of the vital necessity of this book, we knew we couldn't write it alone. We had plenty of questions, but being women, we didn't have all the answers and, equally important, the insights. For these, we needed someone who had walked in the wing-tips, the work boots, the loafers, the tennis shoes, the bedroom slippers, and even the bare feet of a diabetic man. We needed, in short, a multi-faceted diabetic man himself and one with the expertise as well as the life experience to give authoritative answers and give them with empathy and compassion. Namely, we needed Peter A. Lodewick, M.D., endocrinologist, diabetologist, author of *A Diabetic Doctor Looks at Diabetes: His and Yours*, and a diabetic for 23 years.

Fortunately for us and for you diabetic men and you women in their lives, we all got what we needed.

Introduction

by Peter A. Lodewick, M.D.

When June and Barbara approached me about writing this book, I was stunned. Who, me? Why me? With all the great men out there—statesmen, star athletes, creative artists, captains of industry—who live their lives with diabetes, why should I be chosen to explain the impact of this disease on men's lives? But then as I considered it more carefully, it became apparent. Diabetes had struck me in the prime of my life. I'd just completed the grueling years of medical school and medical internship and was coasting happily along serving my country in the U.S. Navy. Although it was the Vietnam year of 1968, I was stationed homeside at the Washington Naval Base when my diabetes was first diagnosed. Oddly enough, this was the most tranquil and least stressful period of my life. My duty as a General Medical Officer was free and easy—8:00 A.M. to 4:30 P.M. with a 2-hour lunch break. Here I was, contemplating reaping the benefits of all the hard labor I had put into accomplishing my lifelong dream of becoming a doctor, when I was hit hard by the diagnosis of diabetes.

As I reflect back on it, I'm sure that either unconsciously or consciously I felt at times that diabetes was an attack on me as a man. Before I could even accept the *possibility* that I had diabetes, I rationalized a lot. Even my typical and intense symptoms of high blood sugar—extreme thirst (although in my beer-drinking days of college I couldn't guzzle beer, I now found myself guzzling large quantities of plain, spiritless water), excessive urination and getting up several times at night for trips to the bathroom, fatigue, and weight loss—couldn't convince me that I was diabetic. I foolishly ignored these symptoms for months. I told myself repeatedly that no one as healthy as I had always been could possibly have diabetes. There was no diabetes in my very large family, including parents, uncles, cousins, and forefathers. More immediately, my four brothers and I were of unusually healthy stock. We were never sick. Not only that, but we would take on any challenge in the Brooklyn neighborhood where we grew up and considered ourselves invincible on the basketball court and in all the numerous other sports we engaged in. I told myself that, like my brothers, I was indomitable against any sports rival and similarly impervious to disease.

It was not until I got on the scale after several months of intense symptoms of high blood sugar that reality hit home. My six-foot three-inch frame had dwindled down to 152 pounds. I then knew why my athletic ability had been steadily declining at my still youthful age of 26 years. As a doctor, I was being that much more of a fool to continue denying diabetes any longer. It was no surprise when I discovered that my urine tested positive for sugar. The blood sugar tests shortly afterward corroborated the diagnosis with levels in excess of 400 milligrams of sugar per decaliter of blood (mg/dl) (normal is around 100 mg/dl).

I felt sure that this was the end. I was convinced that all the devastating complications I'd just learned about in medical school would cut my career short. There was no sense in my pursuing a medical degree in ophthalmology, the study and treatment of diseases of the eye, which had been my plan until diabetes struck. I feared that blindness from diabetes would certainly prohibit me from pursuing this field of medicine. I supposed that the stress and long hours involved in many of the other fields of medicine would also be too great a burden and would accelerate the tendency for vascular complications that I imagined I might already be suffering from. My goose was cooked, my career done for! I was miserable and full of self-pity.

That's when my wife, Maureen, stepped in. She helped me come to grips with my condition and to accept it. Knowing me as well as any person possibly could, she didn't think of me as any less of a man just because I had diabetes. In fact, she prodded me on. "Pete," she would say, "where's that old invincible you? You're not going to let a little adversity like diabetes take you down for the count, are you? What happened to that brave man who could take on any challenge? Why did you go to medical school, anyway? Wasn't it to help people with disease, to make them aware of what disease is and allow them to continue living their lives comfortably and happily despite their problem? Now you can be even more capable. As a diabetic yourself, think how much more insight you'll have and how you'll be able to allay the fears of those in similar plights."

Of course, I couldn't argue against such logic. Gradually with my wife's encouragement and the constant assurance that she still loved me, I began to come to my senses. I realized that since I'd been healthy prior to the time when the symptoms suddenly struck, I could still be healthy even though I now had diabetes. I knew I would be able to confront the disease, integrate it into my life, and carry on.

As part of the way to integrate it into my life, I decided to specialize in the treatment of diabetes. Some of my medical colleagues actually suggested that I take up a specialty that would be less stressful and have a more regular schedule, such as dermatology or radiology, but I now looked on diabetes as a challenge rather than a career destroyer. Although the course change from ophthalmology to internal medicine would be a difficult one, I knew this was the career that would suit me best.

As I set off to learn as much as I could about diabetes, I realized that I had a long way to go. My years in medical school hadn't provided me with many of the details of diabetes management. Nutrition and dietary information was not taught. The knowledge of different types of diabetes, how insulin is made, and how to use it properly was nowhere in the curriculum. There was much to learn if I wanted to give my patients the best possible treatment and to help them enjoy their lives with as little interference as possible from their confrontation with diabetes, as well as to work with other physicians so they could do equally well with their patients.

While learning about diabetes as a doctor, I've also learned about it as a diabetic, following many of the same pathways as my patients. This has enabled me to identify with them. I've shared the shock of discovery, the denial, and the unrealistic hope, as the diabetes ameliorates in the remission phase, that the diagnosis could possibly have been a mistake. I've experienced the ensuing battle to stave off the need for insulin in an all-out effort with exercise and the use of oral hypoglycemic agents, as well as the realization that insulin must be taken, first one dose, then, in a quest for perfect control, experiments with multiple injections and insulin pumps. I've faced the tribulations of testing urine and blood sugar, wrestled with the inevitable temptations of luscious foods, and worried over how to make adjustments for sports and exercise and minor illnesses.

To me it has been more than worth the struggle of traveling the road of diabetes. Not only has it increased my professional competence and my ability to give practical insights to my patients who must travel that same road, but it has also given me the dividend of excellent health with no significant complications. As a matter of fact, I've not missed one day of work because of illness, despite long, arduous days and many 24-hour shifts that I've had to work because of emergency medical calls. As I look back over the years since my original diagnosis of diabetes, I can honestly say that it has in no way prevented me from reaching the goals a man most highly desires in life: a successful career balanced with rewarding and restoring leisure activities and enduring personal happiness with a loving wife, family, and friends.

My greatest hope is that the succeeding chapters in this book will, by helping you control this tricky and far from perfectly understood condition of diabetes, enable you to achieve your own personal goals and make your life dreams a reality.

The
PHYSICAL MAN
. . . .

Oh Say Can You C?

In this chapter Dr. Lodewick will explain to you the standard scientific classification of diabetes: Type I, insulin-dependent, and Type II, non-insulin-dependent. As educators in the field of diabetes, we (June, the Type I diabetic, and Barbara, the nondiabetic) have come up with our own less scientific but, we think, equally valid classification. We evolved this original theory a few years ago when we were speaking at a professional seminar at the Eisenhower Medical Center in Palm Desert, California. After giving our talk, we listened to the physician speakers to learn more, as we always do. And as always, again and again we heard many of these professionals recite the dismal statistics about people with diabetes—how they are this percentage more likely to go blind and that percentage more likely to have kidney failure and the other percentage more likely to have one or more feet amputated.

Disgusted at having to listen to this tired old litany of the supposedly inevitable dire consequences of diabetes, June glanced over at diabetic triathlete Bill Carlson, who was seated in the audience near us. He was lean, fit, and glowing with health. He'd been on a bike ride of 110 miles the day before and on his usual long-distance run that very morning. What did these statistics have to do with him?

June thought about herself and the fact that, at her age (mid-60s), she was healthier and in much better shape than all of her nondiabetic contemporaries and even many women 10 or 15 years younger. What did these statistics have to do with her? After 25 years of diabetes, she had zero diabetes complications. Why weren't these doctors talking about people like her and Bill Carlson?

At dinner that night we discussed this situation. June theorized that people should recognize two *new* categories of diabetes: Type C (for controlled) and Type U (for uncontrolled). They are really two different diseases with two different prognoses. All those horror stories many health professionals seem to relish recounting, all those statistics of the supposed inevitable results of diabetes apply only to the Type U's. And these Type U's—as a result of new knowledge and therapies—are a diminishing group, as more and more of them move into the Type C category.

This lack of recognition of the difference between Type C's and Type U's is infuriating to the Type C diabetics who know better. Ron Brown, our former dietitian and now a fourth-year medical student, told us of reading in one of his medical texts the flat statement that "diabetics don't heal well." He threw down the book and growled, "This is not only ridiculous, it's scientifically inaccurate. I heal as well as anybody." And so he does because he's a total Type C.

Wrongly dumping all diabetics into the Type U category can result in some egregious errors in the diagnosis of medical conditions. Once when June was plagued with a painful thumb joint, an orthopedist incorrectly diagnosed her as having diabetic neuropathy. Why? Because he noticed on her chart that she was diabetic, and "of course, all diabetics develop neuropathy." A correct diagnosis from a different physician revealed that what she actually had was an arthritic joint. The arthritis had nothing to do with diabetes. It had been caused by her falling off her bicycle and catching herself on that hand. She ultimately had the joint surgically replaced with a plastic one. The doctor who performed the operation remarked on how quickly she healed after her surgery—"far faster than most of my patients."

This Type U and Type C categorical confusion also exists in the public mind. When the average person knows anything at all about diabetes, it's usually something horrible—and wrong. The publisher of a number of our books on diabetes ironically developed diabetes himself. (And they say it isn't catching!) At any rate, his wife, a multitalented performer, was preparing for a television special, and he decided not to disturb and distract her by telling her about his diagnosis until the broadcast was over.

One morning at breakfast before he revealed his secret, she was musing on how really fortunate they were because they had each other and a wonderful daughter, were successful in their careers, and that "neither of us has one of those terrible diseases like cancer or heart trouble or diabetes."

He gulped. "Well, gee honey, diabetes isn't so bad. There are lots worse things than that."

"Are you kidding? Diabetes is horrible. It makes you go blind and be on dialysis and get your feet cut off and things like that."

Another victim of the Type U versus Type C confusion! Now she knows better. She knows her husband has diabetes and she also knows the significant difference that control will make in his future well-being. It has inspired her to be an active volunteer worker in diabetes to help others learn that difference.

Our idea is that we should all work toward that happy day when every diabetic is a Type C and there's not a Type U to be seen. Then we will never again have to listen to those wretched and boring statistics.

So now we must put the question to you: are you going to join the happy breed of Type C men or are you going to make yourself into a Type U? Unlike with Type I and Type II, where you have no choice in the matter, you *do* have the power to decide whether you will be a Type C or a Type U. You can go either way. Dr. Lodewick and the two of us are going to do everything within our power to make it easy for you to make the right choice. Read on!

—*June and Barbara*

BEFORE YOU BEGIN

This first chapter contains a lot of basic scientific information about diabetes. If you're unfamiliar with the subject, you may find it fairly heavy going. You may even need to re-read certain parts of the chapter until you are certain you have a thorough understanding of the subject. It will, however, be well worth your while to grit your teeth and slog through it all. Your reward will be a solid foundation of knowledge about diabetes upon which to build your health and your life. Another reward will be that you'll then be able to breeze through the rest of the book, which we promise will be more personal, more upbeat, and even more entertaining than you ever thought a book on diabetes could be.

WHAT YOU'LL FIND HERE

TYPE I AND TYPE II DIABETES

CHOOSING A DOCTOR

BLOOD GLUCOSE SELF-TESTING

GLYCOHEMOGLOBIN (HEMOGLOBIN A_1C) TEST

URINE TESTING

KETOACIDOSIS

DIABETES PILLS

INSULIN THERAPY

AUTOMATIC INJECTORS AND PUMPS

HYPOGLYCEMIC (LOW BLOOD SUGAR) REACTIONS

EYES

HYPERTENSION

CHOLESTEROL AND TRIGLYCERIDES

June and Barbara: We've promised that you would explain the scientific classification of diabetes into Type I and Type II. Why don't you tackle that one first, since it's so basic, and then we can get on with what pertains to diabetic men in particular?

Incidentally, all men should know whether they have Type I or Type II diabetes, as there is a BIG difference between them. In fact, in our *The Diabetic's Book: All Your Questions Answered*, we went so far as to say that "some experts theorize that they are two different diseases," although with both types there is the problem of too much sugar in the blood.

Dr. Lodewick: First, let's discuss how diabetes is diagnosed. Normal blood sugar is 60 to 110 mg/dl when a person is fasting and less than 140 mg/dl two hours after eating.* Diabetes is diagnosed when the blood sugar after an eight-hour fast goes above 140 mg/dl or when the blood sugar two hours after eating goes above 200 mg/dl. However, even though you don't diagnose diabetes when fasting blood sugars are 110 to 140 mg/dl or when blood sugars two hours after eating are 140 to 200 mg/dl, you should not consider blood sugars in these ranges as normal or "borderline diabetes," as we'll discuss extensively below. These blood sugars are abnormal and may be present as "prediabetes" for a long time before diabetes can officially be diagnosed.

---

*Blood sugar levels are measured in milligrams of sugar (glucose) per deciliter of blood. A milligram is 1/1000 of a gram; a deciliter is about 3.3 ounces. In scientific literature and in Canada and most of Europe, blood sugar levels are measured in millimoles per liter (mmol/L). To convert mg/dl to mmol/L, divide by 18. For example, a 60 mg/dl blood sugar is 3.3 mmol/L; a 110 mg/dl blood sugar is 6.1 mmol/L; and a 140 mg/dl is 7.7 mmol/L. You will find a conversion chart of mg/dl to mmol/L in Appendix A.

Once diabetes is actually diagnosed, it is generally of two major types—Type I or Type II. Type I is considered to be insulin-dependent and Type II non-insulin-dependent. The differences between the two are striking. Even the suddenness with which diabetes comes on may be related to the type. In Type I there is an abrupt onset with severe symptoms, so that it seems a person goes from being healthy to being sick almost overnight. With Type II, however, there are minimal and subtle symptoms that can go unnoticed for years before a diagnosis is made.

Over a period of months to years, in Type I diabetes, there is a gradual loss of the insulin-producing cells, the beta cells in the pancreas. Insulin by injection is always needed to control the blood sugar once the beta cells are destroyed. There are genetic, viral, and autoimmune factors that are involved, but the exact chain of events that causes this destruction of the beta cells is not yet known. With loss of beta cells and lack of insulin, not only does blood sugar go high, but there is a breakdown of fat and muscle as well as a number of other problems. This results in the characteristically intense symptoms. In my introduction, I told you about my case. I vividly remember these symptoms: raging thirst, frequent urination, hunger and weight loss despite voracious eating, blurred vision, muscle wasting, lethargy, dry skin and mouth, and varying degrees of mental stupor. If no treatment is started, these symptoms can progress to diabetic coma (ketoacidosis, a form of acid poisoning) and even to death if insulin is not given to get the blood sugar level back to where it should be.

Type II diabetes is another story entirely. The beta cells still produce varying amounts of insulin, but there are also varying degrees of resistance to its effect. To get glucose (sugar) into cells, insulin must attach itself to special chemical structures on cells called receptors. In Type II diabetes there are not enough receptors or they don't work right, so the insulin cannot escort the glucose into the cells and properly dispose of it. Consequently, the blood glucose goes high, just as it does in Type I diabetes.

In contrast to Type I diabetes, however, the blood sugar in Type II does not tend to go as high and may not fluctuate as dramatically. Sometimes there are no symptoms at all! Some of the possible symptoms include fatigue, weight gain, blurred vision, tingling and numbness in the feet, skin infections, and slow healing. Since it's possible to ignore or tolerate these symptoms for a long time, complications may already be present at the time of diagnosis.

Years of high blood sugar can accelerate aging of the blood vessels and nervous system. Slowly and insidiously the well-known and rightly feared complications of diabetes—retinopathy (eye damage), neuropathy (nerve damage), cardiovascular disease and heart attacks, kidney failure, and gangrene and amputation—can develop. Despite the different nature of Type I and Type II diabetes, these complications can be equally severe in both types.

At this point, I would like to reassure you that in Type II (non-insulin-dependent) diabetes, blood sugars can frequently be controlled with proper diet, exercise, and possibly diabetic pills (oral hypoglycemics), so that insulin is not needed. Because being overweight is a primary factor in causing Type II diabetes, losing weight often brings blood sugar down to normal, and good diabetes control can be maintained as long as weight is controlled.

A final difference I'd like to mention concerns heredity. There tends to be a much more distinct hereditary factor with Type II diabetes than with Type I. I have seen as many as six brothers or sisters who all have non-insulin-dependent diabetes. This hereditary pattern is much less apparent in insulin-dependent diabetes, although you will occasionally see families in which there is no family history of diabetes suddenly have two or more children with diabetes.

In Appendix B you will find a chart highlighting the major differences between insulin-dependent and non-insulin-dependent diabetes.

June and Barbara: Now let's fit men into the big diabetes picture. We had always heard that more women than men get diabetes, but at an American Diabetes Association conference we were told that in Europe men are now in the majority. It doesn't make much sense that the incidence of diabetes in the sexes would vary from one continent to another, does it? Do you have any up-to-date and accurate statistics on this? Is there a difference between the man to woman ratio for Type I and Type II?

Dr. Lodewick: The statistics on the incidence of diabetes between the sexes vary according to who is doing the survey. In my 20 years as a diabetologist, I've now seen over 3000 patients. Of the last 1000 patients I've seen, 512 of them were women, 488 were men. The incidence of Type I diabetes is probably equal among the sexes. It's not considered a sexually transmitted condition. In the more than 250 children I've seen in my practice, girls and boys are equally affected with Type I diabetes and this carries over to adulthood for Type I diabetics.

Type II diabetes is a different story. Although diabetes is probably not inherited preferentially in women over men, the prevalence of Type II diabetes is higher in women than in men for several reasons. First, for a number of reasons, women generally live at least six years longer than men. Therefore, they have a higher chance of developing diabetes because the likelihood of developing it increases with age. Second, because of differences in their metabolism, women tend to be obese or overweight more often than men. In data collected from the 1987 Risk Factor Surveillance System, it was found that in 32 states over 26% of the women were more than 20% overweight compared to only 18% of the men. As we know, obesity is one of the causes of Type II diabetes.

To help get more definitive information on hereditary and genetic factors involved in the development of diabetes in men and women, a data bank called the Human Biological Data Interchange has been created. The goal of the data bank is to facilitate research into the etiology (causes) of diabetes. For more information concerning this data bank, you can write the National Disease Research Interchange, 2401 Walnut Street, Suite 408, Philadelphia, PA 19103.

June and Barbara: We've always thought that it was more physiologically difficult for women to handle diabetes than men because of menstruation, pregnancy, menopause, and so on, which dramatically affect diabetes control. Are there any ways in which it's more difficult for a man than a woman?

Dr. Lodewick: It *is* true that the tremendous hormonal fluctuations associated with menstruation, pregnancy, and menopause can be a real challenge for good diabetes control in women. But I find that most women can deal with this challenge once they become committed to it. Men are lucky in that they don't have the frequent physiological hormonal changes that result in fluctuating insulin requirements or alter diabetes control.

It's only when the hormonal changes of adolescence take place that diabetes, as well as cholesterol levels, become more difficult to manage. The male hormones directly increase the demands on insulin requirements and adversely affect cholesterol levels. Indirectly, male hormones somehow affect a man's sense of masculinity; a side effect of this is that he tends to downplay risks. For this reason many men ignore the preventive aspects of diabetes management, paying little attention to diet, taking up smoking, and even indulging or overindulging in alcohol. It's this kind of masculine behavior that may make diabetes more difficult for a man. If he could avoid these self-destructive tendencies, then with testing, knowledge, and the desire to succeed, he should be able to cope with diabetes so that it doesn't interfere with his life's goals.

June and Barbara: Do you find any difference between the percentage of women versus the percentage of men who develop complications?

Dr. Lodewick: There's an equal propensity to develop complications. It doesn't matter whether you are male or female. As I've said, in the general population, women live an average of six to eight years longer than their male counterparts. However, when diabetes sets in, general health problems in diabetic women become manifest at a much earlier age than in nondiabetic women. Take heart disease, for example. Whereas in the nondiabetic woman, it's rare to have angina or coronary heart disease before menopause, in the diabetic woman, the protective effect of the premenopausal state is lost. More women with diabetes have significant heart disease in their 30s. The reason is uncertain, but diabetes control, duration of diabetes, and levels of blood lipids (fats such as cholesterol and triglycerides) may all be important factors. I've seen too many young women who have had major complications in their 20s, but they had very poor control. These complications are rare in patients with good control.

The same goes for young men. When major complications occur at a very young age, almost invariably they happen in men who have very poor control. I am immediately reminded of a young man who I saw for the first time at age 18, diabetic only since the age of 13. He had totally ignored his diabetes, indulging heavily in alcohol and drug use, attempting to defy the statistics, denying that he had a problem or that such a way of living would cause any harm. On initial evaluation, significant retinal changes in the eye were evident and vision loss was imminent. Fortunately, this bad news gave him the motivation to change the course of his life. He got better control of his diabetes and the eye changes reversed. Now, at age 33, he's a happily married father without significant complications.

I think again that this is a reminder that men who indulge in risk-taking behavior or who deny that diabetes is a problem for them are likely to develop complications they will come to regret. And these complications are not always reversible, as they were with the young man just described.

June and Barbara: We often hear men say that their doctors have told them they have "just a touch of diabetes" or "borderline diabetes." We've always believed the old saying about diabetes being like pregnancy. You can't be just a little bit pregnant and you can't be just a little bit diabetic.

Dr. Lodewick: Saying such things as "a touch of diabetes" and "borderline diabetes" is probably just the way the doctor attempts to reassure the man that everything is all right and to allay his anxiety that the well-known catastrophes of diabetes are nothing to fear. I acknowledge that allaying unnecessary anxiety is one of the important roles a physician should provide. However, reassurances like these, which leave the diabetic man in ignorance, can be a major mistake that causes the patient to ignore his diabetes and neglect to take preventive measures. Surely, many diabetic men who have only mild sugar elevations and no symptoms may not go on to develop any of the major complications, nor may many diabetic men who "feel great" but have poor blood sugar control. However, for the one too many of such men who go on to develop a heart attack, impotence, gangrene, or blindness, it's not worth taking the risk or chance.

There is even a condition called Syndrome X, in which diabetes and/or high blood sugar are not present but which is probably a prediabetic syndrome. Even though the person may have normal blood sugars, he may have high insulin levels, high cholesterol, high blood pressure, and more of a tendency toward vascular disease. This asymptomatic condition can be reversed through weight loss and exercise. There are also many preventive measures patients with mild blood sugar elevation can take so that it remains a condition with only minimally high blood sugars that will never cause a medical impact or slow a person down from his life's pursuits. Therefore, a physician should no doubt calm a patient's fears. But that's not enough. He or she must also impress upon the patient that he definitely has diabetes or a possible health-threatening condition, educate him and provide the knowledge he needs to take proper care of himself to avoid medical complications.

June and Barbara: You've led us right into the next important question. Just how do you choose the right doctor, and what should you expect from him or her? Many men want to know, as do women, if they should keep their family doctor (internist, general practitioner, or whatever) or go to a diabetes specialist.

Dr. Lodewick: First, I must admit that there are no perfect physicians. (I'm working on it.) But then there are no perfect patients, either. It takes a great deal of understanding on the part of both the physician and the patient to build a relationship that will result in good diabetes control and avoidance of preventable complications. I can tell you, however, exactly what qualities to look for in an ideal physician, and I hope that with this guidance, you will be fortunate enough to connect with one.

The qualities I've found to be most important are (1) depth and currentness of knowledge, (2) thoroughness, (3) commitment of time and accessibility, (4) educating ability, (5) empathy, and (6) willingness to listen and learn. Let's consider these one by one.

1. DEPTH AND CURRENTNESS OF KNOWLEDGE

A physician's knowledge should not be limited to what he or she has learned in a textbook because much of what is printed in textbooks is soon proven false. Also, textbooks are written in general terms and therefore do not necessarily apply to a given individual.

Many doctors are reluctant to use new treatments, and this can work against the patient, too. For instance, although self-testing of blood sugar has been of real practical use since the late 1970s, there are still many physicians who do not recommend it. This is a sure tip-off that the doctor is way behind the times.

Don't be afraid to ask your doctor questions. If your doctor doesn't know the answers, he or she should be humble enough to admit it and search out the answers for your next visit. If the answers cannot be found, you should be referred to another physician who can answer them.

2. THOROUGHNESS

I've had patients come to me for evaluation who have not had a complete physical examination in years. Some even appeared stunned that I suggested one was needed. A good physician is thorough. This means checking your heart for silent heart disease (even when there are no symptoms), your blood pressure, your eyes for eye damage (even when there is no vision loss), and your feet for signs of neuropathy. You may need a chemistry screen profile, such as my own, which is presented in the Afterword.

3. COMMITMENT OF TIME AND ACCESSIBILITY

This is a tough one. Physicians are always pressed for time because of medical emergencies and acute medical problems. They are not necessarily "playing on the golf course," as many of my patients facetiously suggest. It seems we rarely have enough time to sit and discuss problems or answer questions that people with diabetes have. Yet, the proper management of diabetes takes time, and a physician treating diabetes should spend much more time than is usual in communicating with patients.

As for accessibility, of all the diseases in medicine, I think the one in which the doctor's accessibility is needed most is diabetes. When things go wrong—and they can suddenly, even with the best of self-care—a doctor's 24-hour accessibility is a great source of relief and comfort to the patient. For example, in times of illness when nausea, vomiting, and fever occur and during insulin reactions, the doctor must help you through the emergency and suggest changes in insulin dose before things get worse. Likewise, if you have a condition such as a swollen foot, you need to be able to get prompt medical attention. You should always feel free to call your doctor, even in cases of a false alarm.

4. EDUCATING ABILITY

Since men like having control of their own destiny and do not like leaving it totally in the hands of their doctors, you need to learn as much about diabetes as you can. Therefore, you should look for a physician who has good teaching ability. It's estimated that it takes 30 to 40 hours to educate a person on all aspects of control—what it is and how to gain it. An educated diabetic is one who is totally aware of the consequences of neglect of diabetes and is not carrying around in his head the false message that "I am just a borderline diabetic." Neither is an educated diabetic afraid of possible complications, as he knows they are preventable with proper self-care.

A good physician does not necessarily do all the teaching himself or herself. He or she may enlist the aid of a team of health professionals, including a diabetes nurse-educator or a Certified Diabetes Educator (CDE), a dietitian, a psychotherapist, and possibly even a physical therapist. Or the doctor may suggest a teaching program at a hospital or diabetes treatment center for you to attend. You may be given a reading list of good books. And finally, you may be put in touch with the American Diabetes Association (see Appendix C; for the Canadian Diabetes Association, see Appendix D) and the Juvenile Diabetes Foundation, all of which offer information and publications of importance to your continuing education. (The Juvenile Diabetes Association International is at 432 Park Avenue South, New York, NY 10016-8013 or telephone 1-800-223-1138.)

5. EMPATHY

Empathy means identifying with the feelings and thoughts of another person. Since I, too, have diabetes, I have no trouble with this one, but many physicians do. They can't accept the fact, which I know too well, that our present treatments are too imprecise for anyone to attain constantly perfect blood sugar control. They, therefore, chastise the diabetic and accuse him of "cheating" when blood sugars go high. This criticism is often unfair and you are right to resent it. You can't work with a physician who has this attitude, and it's best to find someone more empathetic.

6. WILLINGNESS TO LISTEN AND LEARN

A physician should have the humility to learn from his or her patients. I've been fooled innumerable times into thinking that my patients needed insulin, when they knew better and refused to take it, and it turned out they were right. In fact, in many instances, after failing on my course of treatment, I listened to my patient's suggestions and they did better following their own advice. No matter how learned a physician is, he or she cannot possibly know you as well as you know yourself. Remember that old medical school adage, "the patient knows best," and expect your doctor to remember it, too, and at least be receptive to your ideas. Finally, most important of all, a good doctor should always provide you with hope and encouragement. You have a right to rely on your doctor to provide these.

Now, if your family doctor is living up to these criteria, I say fine. You're in good hands. But if you're not getting this kind of care and attention, then it's wise to see another doctor, perhaps a diabetes specialist who can and will help you achieve the best of control along with a positive mental attitude.

June and Barbara: We know you are your own doctor in the literal sense of the word, but we read in your first book *A Diabetic Doctor Looks at Diabetes: His and Yours* that you think *every* man who has diabetes must be his own doctor.

Dr. Lodewick: When you first think about it, it might seem a little arrogant for a diabetic man to consider himself capable of being his own doctor. After all, physicians have spent long years in medical school studying to learn about the disease so that they can help their patients. Following this thinking, a patient by comparison is "ignorant" and should heed the advice of his physician, respecting his or her wisdom and authority. However, you must realize that no amount of medical knowledge accumulated through books about the disease can be completely applicable to you as an individual diabetic. You have far too many unique qualities that are beyond the scope of any doctor, no matter how brilliant or resourceful he or she may be. No doctor can know all the peculiarities, the stresses, the diet, the ups and downs, and the conflicts that beset you every day. In addition, the doctor is so busy solving emergencies and urgent crises that he or she is seldom available to spend all the time you may need or want when things go wrong. Nor does the doctor have the time to motivate you to take good care of yourself. Keeping these facts in mind, you will quickly realize that you *must* be your own doctor and strive to gain the knowledge and information you need to give yourself good diabetes self-care.

No matter how well you take care of yourself, though, you'll still need to make regular visits to your physician for physical examinations and to review what things you're doing right and wrong. After all, even the most learned doctors consult with their colleagues.

June and Barbara: It would help if you could give men a review of exactly what good diabetes self-care is so that they can be sure their doctor is doing the job right.

Dr. Lodewick: Good self-care simply means keeping your blood sugar as near to normal as possible. Diet, exercise, insulin, stress, and travel are a few of the factors that affect the control of blood sugar, and in the rest of the book we'll deal with these separately. Since each of us is unique, these factors affect each man differently. Even if a physician sees you regularly, these effects are difficult to determine except by the diabetic man himself. After all, you have diabetes 24 hours a day, and you have to be a 24-hour-a-day caretaker. You must evaluate your own symptoms and, in that sense, assume the role of being your own doctor. Although some men may not think of themselves as competitive, in my opinion all people are competitive in that they desire to do their best. That's where setting goals may help. Set goals for the blood sugar levels you would like to attain. Ideally, you should aim for levels of 70 to 140 mg/dl before meals and 100 to 160 mg/dl after eating. By setting these blood sugar goals, you have an incentive to do the tests that will help you analyze the factors that affect control. Then make the appropriate changes in those areas to ensure that you are reaching the goals you set.

Likewise, to ensure the best outcome for health, it is also important to set goals for the number of calories you eat, for body weight, for blood cholesterol levels, and for the amount of exercise you do. What these different goals should be will differ from person to person, but by relying on his competitive spirit, a man can better achieve his goals. We will discuss goals for calories, weight, cholesterol, and exercise as we proceed through the chapters of this book.

Your methods of self-care will vary depending on whether you have insulin-dependent (Type I) or non-insulin-dependent (Type II) diabetes. Type I men need to understand insulin, how long each type lasts, when it "peaks" (is most powerful), and how to alter the dosage depending on their blood sugar. Most of you Type I men should be taking more than one shot a day for optimum control. You Type II men should keep your weight at an ideal level. Some of you need to take pills to lower your blood sugar (oral hypoglycemics), and you must learn how to use these properly.

All of you, whether Type I or Type II, have to learn to control your eating and know how much food you need depending on your weight, exercise level, and medication, if any. You must set exercise goals and stick to them. It's not too uncommon for someone to come home from work dog-tired and decide to put off until tomorrow taking a run or getting on the rowing machine. However, even if you set a goal starting with as little as a one-fourth or one-half mile walk per day, you'll eventually reach your best as you shoot for higher and higher goals.

June and Barbara: When you were first diagnosed diabetic in 1968, testing your urine for its sugar content was the only way to have any idea whether your diabetes was in control or not. June was diagnosed in 1967, and she, too, was told by her doctor to test her urine and report the negative or positive results. However, while we were writing our *Diabetic's Sports & Exercise Book* in 1976, some diabetic sportsmen alerted us to the procedure of blood sugar testing. June immediately borrowed a meter from a representative of the manufacturer and started testing her blood sugar. Though her urine tests had been largely negative over the years, her blood sugar tests stunned us. She was not in control at all, and this proved to us once and for all the deceptive nature of testing urine for sugar. We've been passionate advocates of blood sugar testing ever since.

We noticed in your book, *A Diabetic Doctor Looks at Diabetes: His and Yours*, that you had some positive points to make about urine testing. Which method of testing do you favor now and why?

Dr. Lodewick: It's no contest. There's no doubt that blood sugar testing is by far the superior method. Ask a diabetes specialist or any physician who treats many diabetes patients. The vast majority rely on blood sugar testing in the hospital setting to get diabetes under control and start their patients on self-testing of blood sugar at home so they can make fine-tuning adjustments in their diet, insulin, and exercise.

One recent case I had demonstrates the value of blood sugar testing. A 62-year-old gentleman with diabetes of many years' duration thought he was doing well, especially when his urine tests were negative. He hated the inconvenience and expense of blood sugar testing and he particularly hated the discomfort of the spring-loaded devices for puncturing his fingers. When his glycohemoglobin test (a laboratory test for overall blood sugar control) came back at 12.4%, (normal is below 8%), he protested, showing me his urine test book, in which most of the results were excellent.

We then proceeded to take a blood sugar test simultaneously with a urine sugar test. The urine test was negative. The blood sugar test showed his blood sugar was 282 mg/dl. He was impressed—and convinced.

This man had a high renal threshold. This means that his kidneys don't spill sugar into the urine until the blood sugar gets very high—in some people this can be well over 250 mg/dl, as was probably the case with this man and also with June. For these people, "good" urine tests may not reflect good control.

Then there is the reverse: the low renal threshold. This is when the kidneys spill sugar into the urine even when blood sugars are in the normal range. The most obvious example of this is during pregnancy. (Don't worry, men, you won't have this problem!) As many as 50% of pregnant women spill sugar into their urine despite having normal blood sugars. Young people and children also commonly have low renal thresholds. Since their blood sugar could be anywhere from 60 to 400 mg/dl, in spite of sugar in the urine, you can't change insulin dose or diet based on their urine test result.

There is even a problem when the renal threshold is at the average of 180 mg/dl (normal threshold) because the urine is reflecting the blood sugar of the preceding several hours and not what it is at the moment of the test. In other words, with urine testing you never know exactly what your blood sugar is at any given time. Theoretically, you can get a partial idea of your blood sugar at a particular time by first emptying your bladder of the urine that has accumulated over the preceding several hours. Then you let urine collect in your bladder for the next half hour (called the second voided specimen) and test it. If the urine now tests negative, you can then presume that your blood sugar is in a reasonably good range under 180 mg/dl. If it is positive, you can presume that your blood sugar is slightly over 180 mg/dl. But even following this procedure, you can't use an extra dose of insulin to fine-tune diabetes control, as you could if you had tested your blood sugar. On the other hand, if your urine tests are negative four times a day and your glyco-hemoglobin is normal, urine testing may suffice for you.

One problem that can interfere with proper interpretation of the results of the second voided urine test occurs when you have an inability to empty your bladder completely. When this happens, it's impossible to get a second void. There are numer-ous conditions that can cause this: spinal cord injuries, multiple sclerosis, strokes, aging, diabetic neuropathy, and an enlarged prostate, a common condition in men that blocks urine outflow.

All too often I have seen patients make the mistake of giving themselves extra insulin based on high urine sugar, only to provoke insulin reactions. What happens is that blood sugar can be 60 mg/dl when the urine sugar is very high, the urine having collected sugar over the preceding several hours. For some reason, people who do this will not listen when I tell them that there's no way their urine test results can be precise. They repeatedly try to clear the urine of sugar with extra insulin, and they repeatedly have more insulin reactions. They are the "doubting Thomases" of the diabetic world. Thank goodness self-testing of blood sugar came along, and now they can *know* when they do or do not need extra insulin.

June and Barbara: We agree with you wholeheartedly that blood sugar testing easily proves itself more precise and accurate than urine testing. Could you now explain how blood sugar testing gives a diabetic man the self-education he needs so that he can make adjustments in insulin, diet, exercise, and stress levels to improve control?

Dr. Lodewick: Testing is what gives you the knowledge you must have to help you decide what blood sugar goals to shoot for. It allows you to understand the factors that cause blood sugar to go up or down and, consequently, to make appropriate changes in your treatment plan. You'll see, for instance, that certain foods cause your blood sugar to go high despite the fact that you are not "cheating on your diet," as your doctor may have wrongly accused you of. That's because different foods, although they may contain the same number of calories and carbohydrates, can cause different rises in blood sugar. This is called the "glycemic index" of foods (see Appendix G). For example, cooked carrots will raise blood sugar twice as much as the same amount of cooked peas even though they may be equal on the American Diabetes Association Exchange Lists for Meal Planning, the standard eating guide for diabetics.

In addition, foods listed on the ADA Exchange Lists are only approximately equivalent in the amount of carbohydrates. (Carbohydrates raise blood sugar more than proteins or fat and therefore must be watched more carefully.) When measurements for breads, for instance, are given in household terms rather than ounces or grams, you can get more than you bargained for. Daisy Kuhn, a California microbiology professor, has made many diabetics aware of this with the poem she wrote about bagels. (A starch/bread exchange on the Exchange Lists is supposed to be 15 grams of carbohydrate. One-half of a bagel, one ounce, is listed as one starch/bread exchange.)

THE BAGEL
The bagel is delicious,
Its weight can be capricious.
With onion, poppy seeds, or spice,
A bagel you must slice.
The biggest from the Bagel Nosh
Weighed 4.5 ounces, by gosh!
So get out your scale
To make yourself hale.
It's the grams of carbohydrate that count,
Not the bread exchange—half a bagel!

Dr. Kuhn explains that one-half of her bagel would have been over *two* bread exchanges, or nearly 34 grams of carbohydrate.

In addition to food insights, testing is also crucial if you're an athlete to help you know your best performance blood sugar level and how to achieve it. This will be discussed in more detail in Chapter 4. Briefly though, many athletes I've spoken to feel that they perform better when their blood sugar level right before heavy exercise starts out slightly high—in the range of 120 to 200 mg/dl. The only way you can find out what range you're in is by self-testing.

Finally, as so many people realize, stress plays a big role in diabetes control. Self-testing is a way of seeing the effect of stress. This reminds me of a story told by Dr. Lois Jovanovic-Peterson in *The Diabetic Woman*. She had a female patient who had tested her blood sugar at 9:00 A.M. one morning and found it normal. Then her dog, to whom she was very attached, suddenly died. At 10:00 A.M., without having eaten anything, her blood sugar soared to 300 mg/dl. This is a classic example of what stress does to diabetics. Throughout this book, we will detail the significant role stress plays in diabetes control—in the workplace and in family situations and life circumstances.

June and Barbara: We've certainly seen this stress phenomenon in June's life. When she is under stress, her blood sugar can go up 75 mg/dl in 15 minutes. It often happens to people when they go to the doctor. Say you take your blood sugar at home and it's normal; then when you have it taken in the doctor's office, it's over 200. This may lead you to believe that your home blood sugar meter is reading low or not working right. In reality, what you've experienced is the "white coat syndrome," which are the symptoms you get when you go to the doctor's office. It's recently been discovered that many people are falsely diagnosed as having high blood pressure simply because being in the presence of a doctor has frightened them into temporary hypertension. The same thing can happen to your blood sugar. And the emotion isn't always fear. Anger—at having to wait so long, at the anticipated bill, or at some remark the doctor makes—can be just as destructive. Your blood sugar tests can be a vivid record of the course of your emotions.

Since stress and other factors can wreak their havoc on Type II's as well as Type I's, we should ask next if you generally recommend blood sugar testing to your Type II's. It has been our observation that many of them are told by their doctors that since they have a "mild" case of diabetes, they don't need to bother testing at home.

Dr. Lodewick: I always recommend blood sugar self-testing to my Type II patients. They definitely *do* need to test. If they are unable to get consistently normal blood sugars, then they can find out why. Is the glycemic index playing a role? Are they eating extra large bagels that raise their blood sugar even though there's no sugar in them? Is it lack of exercise or too much stress—the usual factors that can affect the sugar level? The following is an example of a man with Type II diabetes who found blood sugar testing invaluable when he wanted to keep from having to take insulin.

MAN WARDS OFF INSULIN

Ed, a 58-year-old RCA engineer, had had diabetes for more than five years. Initially, he was satisfied that he could control it when he normalized his blood sugar with diet and a 20-pound weight loss. But then he got sloppy. He knew he wasn't doing well, but didn't want to believe it. Over the ensuing years, his weight climbed and his blood sugars increasingly rose. My repeated admonitions did nothing to cause him to make changes. Finally, he reached the depths of metabolic and diabetes control, as reflected in these numbers:

August 1, 1989

Glycohemoglobin	14.4% (normal: 4.2 to 8.2%, Metpath Labs)
Weight	220 lbs (normal: 175 lbs)
Cholesterol	256 mg/dl (normal: less than 200 mg/dl)
Blood sugar	311 mg/dl (normal: less than 140 mg/dl)
Triglycerides	456 mg/dl (normal: less than 200 mg/dl)

In the face of these terrible test results, we drew up an agreement: if he couldn't improve his control significantly in the next four weeks, he would begin taking insulin. I suggested he test his blood sugar four times a day, and if his blood sugars were over 120 mg/dl, then he should omit most of his heavy carbohydrates.

At first things didn't look too hopeful. During the initial few days of blood sugar recordings, *all* his blood sugar tests were over 200 mg/dl, with a few over 300 mg/dl. The highest was 347 mg/dl. Six weeks later there was a tendency toward improvement, but he still had very little control: average blood sugar was 164 mg/dl, and 20% of the tests were still above 233 mg/dl, with the highest again at 347 mg/dl. But after six more weeks of conscientious effort, his average blood sugar was 97 mg/dl, with the highest only 180 mg/dl. As a result of such dramatic improvement, he was rewarded with the following test results:

October 15, 1989

Glycohemoglobin	9.2
Weight	184 lbs
Cholesterol	178 mg/dl
Blood sugar	78 mg/dl
Triglycerides	153 mg/dl

There was no need for insulin for this RCA engineer. In his own words: "Blood sugar testing is the answer."

June and Barbara: This is beginning to sound like an unqualified endorsement of blood sugar testing. We find that in most areas of life, there is usually a downside. Is this true about blood sugar testing? Are there any circumstances that would make it deceiving or undesirable in any way?

Dr. Lodewick: Yes, I've seen blood sugar tests boomerang and lead to bad rather than good control in some Type II patients who've gone into a protracted period of remission with normal blood sugars after initial treatment. After diet and other measures bring their blood sugars back to normal, some Type II men may produce more of their own insulin and will react to it better. I've seen many such men, relieved to see their blood sugars normal again, begin thinking that maybe their diabetes diagnosis is a mistake. Then they start experimenting and falling into careless habits. When they try a donut, test their blood sugar, and find that it stays normal, they feel they can continue to indulge in high-calorie delights full of fat and sugar. Eventually, their weight balloons and their risk of heart disease, high blood sugar, and high cholesterol increases. Their diabetes again gets out of control and may not be as easy to get back in control the second time around. On the other hand, I've also seen Type II men keep their blood sugars normal for more than 30 years.

June and Barbara: Taking daily blood sugar tests at home is, of course, the secret of good diabetes therapy, but there's another test that can give a man a valuable overall assessment of his diabetes control. This is the glycohemoglobin test we mentioned earlier. (It is also known as the hemoglobin A_1C test.) June likes this test because it makes her feel good to know that she is in the normal range, and so far she has been. Could you enlighten our readers about this test and explain why they should have one on a regular basis?

Dr. Lodewick: The glycohemoglobin level is a very important blood test in the study and treatment of diabetes. What it tells you is how well diabetes is controlled over a six- to ten-week period. If measurements are made on diabetics every eight weeks, this may, from a research standpoint, answer the important question of whether good to excellent control of diabetes means fewer medical complications than poor control. Doctors think it does, but until this test became available, we could not document which patients had good control versus those who had poor control (doctors could only suspect those with poor control).

As an example, I know one young man in particular whom I suspected of having poor control, but I could never prove it because when he came in for his blood sugar test, he would invariably get a normal result between 70 and 110 mg/dl. He would deny that his blood sugars were poor between visits, so I could never urge him to improve his control. Finally, the glycohemoglobin test became available. My young friend's glycohemoglobin was 14 to 15%—*twice the normal level!* Although I could have used this information as a club, I just let him know that his control was not very good between doctor's visits. I reassured him that if he knew how to get his blood sugars normal for his office visits, he had the knowledge to get better control between visits as well, which would do much to preserve his good looks. He responded well to this encouragement.

How close to a normal glycohemoglobin level should a man aim for? This depends. For a Type II diabetic who does not require insulin, I would definitely try for perfect control, that is, a normal level. If your test falls in the normal range, this means less demand on your beta cells to secrete insulin and, consequently, less chance of non-insulin-dependent diabetes turning into insulin-dependent.

Type I diabetes is a somewhat different story. The techniques we now have for normalizing blood sugars, and thus glycohemoglobin, are far from perfect. Unlike insulin secreted by the pancreas, insulin injected with a needle does not absorb consistently (the speed with which it is absorbed can even change depending on the site of injection). This means it's virtually impossible for even the most conscientious of Type I's to maintain ideal blood sugar levels all the time. And if they work too hard at never having high blood sugar, they run the risk of more frequent low blood sugars and this can be dangerous because insulin reactions can result in bizarre behavior and unconsciousness. It has been shown in the Diabetes Control and Complications Trial, a major National Institutes of Health study, that the risk of hypoglycemia is three times as high in those shooting for perfect control. Therefore, it's probably adequate for Type I's to settle for glycohemoglobins in the fair to good range, rather than normal.

I should mention that the normal range depends on how the laboratory does the test. Be sure to find out what that range is for the particular laboratory your physician uses. My laboratory, Metpath, has the following ranges for glycohemoglobin: normal is 4 to 8.2%, fair diabetes control is 8.2 to 9.2%, and poor diabetes control is 9.2 to 18%.

June and Barbara: We haven't said many good things about urine testing here. Can you tell us any reasons why urine testing still might be useful?

Dr. Lodewick: Economics, for one. Urine testing is much cheaper. I don't know why blood sugar test strips cost so much more than urine test strips, but they do (65¢ versus 8¢). Also, urine testing is much simpler, especially for men, although it may cause other men in public restrooms to wonder what you're up to. All you have to do is pass a urine test strip through the urinary stream, and by the time you're zipped up and out the door, you'll know the amount of sugar in your urine. Finally, there are men who simply cannot stand the sight of blood. They may use urine testing as a very weak alternative to blood testing.

June and Barbara: The good news is that before long there may be a way for everyone—bloodophobes included—to test their blood sugar without having to stick their fingers or see blood. We recently received this press release:

> INDIANA, PA—June 25, 1990—Biocontrol Technology, Inc. (NASDAQ:BICO), a developer and manufacturer of biomedical devices, announced today that the company will have a working prototype of its new noninvasive glucose sensor in August of this year. Management at the company said the device is a major breakthrough in the management of diabetes, a disease that afflicts 70 million persons worldwide.
>
> To make life easier for diabetics, the company's sensor will measure glucose levels simply by being held against a person's

skin, replacing the current method of finger pricking for blood glucose testing. The device operates by emitting a flow of energy directly into the patient's body tissue. The sensing device registers numerically how the energy flow interacts with the tissue, indicating the glucose level in the body. An unlimited number of readings could be taken daily, according to the company, since no blood sampling is required.

Two models of the glucose sensor are planned. The first model, scheduled to be put into production at the company's Indiana, Pa, facility in late 1990 or early 1991, is a desktop unit appropriate for clinical use. A smaller, more portable device for patient self-testing will go into production late in 1991.

Diasense, Inc., a subsidiary of Biocontrol also located in Indiana, Pa, will coordinate the marketing of the device.

Before we leave the subject of the infamous finger stick, we should also report that writing in the *New England Journal of Medicine*, Dr. Steven Grenell of Montefiore Medical Center in the Bronx urges diabetics to stick themselves in the thigh or forearm when they do home blood sugar tests. He said, "The fingertip is one of the most sensitive areas of the body, but as far as is known capillary blood glucose content is everywhere equal."

Barbara, not being a diabetic who has to take multiple blood sugars, was willing to be the guinea pig for this. Pressing as hard as possible on the inside of her forearm with the blood-letting device, she pressed the button. Only a minute drop came out despite repeated squeezing. She tried again in a different spot, but with no more success. The result was one bruise and one black spot on her arm—and not enough blood to do the test. June pointed out that even if there had been a rather hearty drop of blood, it couldn't be used in some of the meters, for example, the One Touch, for which you have to apply the blood directly into the meter.

There have been other theories of places where you can get blood for the test—the toes, if you first ascertain that there is sufficient circulation not to run any risk of infection; the ear lobe, which is another place where it would be a little difficult to get the blood into a One Touch; and the penis. On that painful note, let us return to urine testing and when it is effective, or at least not too ineffective.

Dr. Lodewick: In particular, urine testing could be used for the newly diabetic patient after his blood sugar has been normalized by whatever means are necessary—insulin, pills, diet, and/or exercise. Once your blood sugar is stabilized, there's no sense testing blood sugar four or five times a day if you find it is always normal. Urine testing or spot checking of blood sugar could be used to make sure you're staying normal in this remission phase. (This phase is also called the "honeymoon" phase because, although it can last for an indefinite period of time, it always does come to an end.) As long as blood sugars remain normal, and this is confirmed by a good long-term glycohemoglobin check, all is fine. If the urine becomes positive, more frequent testing or a return to blood sugar testing is in order.

June and Barbara: We haven't mentioned the most important reason for testing urine—not for determining what your blood sugar is, but to see if you have ketones, those sinister calling cards of out-of-control diabetes. Could you tell us more about ketones and when men should test for them?

Dr. Lodewick: To understand ketones, it's important to realize that insulin doesn't just let sugar into the cells to provide the energy to run the body. It also has an effect on muscle and fat metabolism, as mentioned earlier. When there's not enough insulin or when the cells aren't using it properly, not only does the blood sugar build up, but the body begins to break down its own fat and muscle in an attempt to provide the energy needed to keep functioning. This breakdown forms acidic toxins, or ketones, resulting in what is variously called *acidosis, ketosis, ketoacidosis*, or most vividly, *acid poisoning*. This condition can be life-threatening. It's estimated that 5 to 15% of diabetics who develop ketoacidosis will die from it if they don't do something about it fast. But take heart; you can almost always avoid this condition.

I've seen patients who were hospitalized as many as five times a year with ketoacidosis. One man had to go to the hospital with it *20 times* in one year. But after coming under my care, he finally learned how to prevent it and he never had to go to the hospital with ketoacidosis again. I'd like to think of myself as the hero who overcame the problem that nobody else could solve, but all I did was to give him some basic information and motivate him to be more attentive to his diabetes.

June and Barbara: What is this basic information on keto-acidosis that will keep men free from this potentially life-threatening condition?

Dr. Lodewick: First, ketoacidosis is caused by insulin defi-ciency. Therefore, you Type II diabetic men don't need to worry about it since you usually have high levels of blood insulin. It's possible, however, that some of you who were initially diag-nosed as being non-insulin-dependent may eventually develop insulin-dependent diabetes, especially if you have a serious illness. Therefore, it's important for both Type I's and Type II's to understand the insidious chain of events that lead to ketoacidosis.

When you don't have enough insulin, the sugar in your blood cannot be escorted across cell membranes where it can be used for energy or stored. Thus, your blood sugar goes up. What's worse, your blood sugar then proceeds to go even higher by a process called *gluconeogenesis*, which simply means new formation of glucose. This takes place in the liver when there's an insulin deficiency. It's important for you to remember this because it explains why your blood sugar can get high even when you don't eat or drink anything. This is also the reason why you Type I diabetic men should usually not stop taking your insulin even if you have nausea and vomiting and can't hold food down.

As your blood sugar goes ever higher and higher, your kidneys can't absorb all the sugar and so it spills into the urine.

Your body tries to get rid of this excess sugar in the urine by taking more water from the bloodstream to increase urination. This, in turn, makes the body dehydrated, which makes you increasingly thirsty. If you try to quench your thirst with something that contains calories such as orange juice or milk, this makes your blood sugar go even higher and further increases your urination, thirst, and dehydration. And the vicious cycle goes on and on.

Other symptoms that accompany insulin deficiency and/or high blood sugar include blurred vision, muscle weakness, fatigue, lethargy, irritability, and interrupted sleep because of the constant urination and vomiting. You are also likely to be losing body minerals such as sodium, potassium, phosphorus, and possibly calcium.

I must emphasize, however, that you can have high blood sugar and some of these symptoms of insulin deficiency *without* having ketoacidosis. Over a long period of time, high blood sugar can bring on the classic *chronic* complications of diabetes, but there is no immediate, life-threatening *acute* danger without acidosis.

You become prone to acidosis when you have a more severe insulin deficiency and, since sugar can't get into the cells to provide fuel for the body and brain, the body, in its desperate need for fuel, starts breaking down its own fat. (This also takes place in the liver.) The by-products of the fat breakdown, ketoacids or ketones, are what cause the acidosis—an acid condition in the blood. This acidity, along with high blood sugar, dehydration, and mineral deficiency, affects the function of the cells. If this condition is serious enough, it can lead to death.

Barbara and June: Since ketoacidosis is such a sinister condition, tell us when it is most likely to occur so that Type I diabetic men can be on the alert for it.

Dr. Lodewick: There are six potential ketoacidic situations.

1. When you don't take your regular dose (or doses) of insulin.

2. When you are a new diabetic and you don't realize that your body doesn't have enough insulin.

3. When you overeat or overdrink, especially high-calorie drinks such as milk, juice, beer, or soda. This may cause you to become relatively insulin deficient even though you are taking your regular doses of insulin.

4. When you are sick. Even a minor illness can increase the demand for insulin so that you need more to overcome the insulin resistance that develops with an illness. If vomiting occurs for more than four hours, you must make sure that you don't have ketoacidosis.

5. When you are under severe emotional stress. This is particularly common in teenagers when puberty and the struggle for self-sufficiency can cause hormonal changes that can make them relatively insulin deficient and therefore more susceptible to ketoacidosis.

6. I have not personally seen this in patients, but it is reported that heavy exercise in patients with poorly controlled diabetes can actually aggravate the diabetic state rather than improve it.

June and Barbara: The obvious answer, then, is to test for ketones in the urine under any of these circumstances. In fact, June prudently tests for them any time she finds her blood sugar over 200 mg/dl in two consecutive tests.

Dr. Lodewick: That's not a bad idea. If you do find ketones in your urine, especially if you have been vomiting for more than four hours, you should inform your doctor so you can work together on increasing your insulin dose to prevent or alleviate this potentially life-threatening condition. (This is one time when you shouldn't rely on being your own doctor.) Review with your doctor how you can take extra insulin when your blood sugar is high and you have ketones in your urine.

June and Barbara: How do you test for ketones?

Dr. Lodewick: You make the test with Chemstrips K or Ketostix. Just follow the simple instructions that come in the package. You can also test for ketones with Chemstrips uGK and Keto-Diastix, which also test for sugar in your urine.

June and Barbara: A woman we know who started working as a receptionist in a diabetes center noticed a strange phenomenon. Many of the patients had an extremely unpleasant odor about them. It didn't matter if the patients were young or old, male or female, the odor was identical. It was not the standard body odor associated with sweat or uncleanliness, but an overwhelming, sickening aura of overripe fruit. She later realized this was the "acetone breath" smell of out-of-control diabetes. She said it didn't seem to come from any specific part of their bodies, but it surrounded them like a heavy, portable fog. Not only were these people well on the road to diabetes complications, they were making themselves socially unacceptable to uninformed people. (Actually, even an informed person would have trouble accepting a constant barrage of this noxious odor.)

It would seem that any man striving for success in a career couldn't afford to carry such an offensive handicap around with him. Even if he weren't willing to keep his blood sugar in control to prevent long-term complications, he might be willing to do it to keep potential employers, colleagues, and clients from fleeing from the room when he came in.

Dr. Lodewick, have you noticed this noxious diabetic aroma in many of your patients? If so, did you tell them about it, and did it give some of them the impetus to control their diabetes when nothing else seemed to work?

Dr. Lodewick: From the strictly medical standpoint, there are several odors that can come from diabetes. The one you mentioned, the fruity odor generated from the breath or mouth, comes from very out-of-control diabetes with some degree of ketoacidosis. Generally, the diabetes has to be moderately to severely out of control for this to happen. With this degree of poor control, usually the man is too sick to carry his workload, especially if it's a difficult load.

Sometimes poor diabetes control without ketoacidosis can cause changes in the skin, including dryness, cracking, and even fungus and yeast infections. These may lead to very bad odors. Good diabetes control along with skin and genital care will prevent this. There is also an offensive odor that is associated with kidney failure. This is caused by the release of toxins through the lungs. Again, good diabetes control will prevent kidney failure and the odor it causes.

June and Barbara: While we're on the topic of insulin deficiency, would you say that people who take insulin have more serious diabetes than those who don't?

Dr. Lodewick: No. People tend to equate taking insulin with serious diabetes, and if they take more than one dose of insulin in a day, they think it's even worse. What they don't realize is that taking insulin is only a way of getting control of blood sugar. Often it's actually easier to get better control with 3 or 4 doses of insulin per day than it is with just one dose. In addition, some people taking over 100 units of insulin frequently don't need any. These are Type II's who are overweight. Their excess weight makes them resistant to their own insulin and to any insulin they may be taking by injection. By losing weight and going on a low-calorie diet, they can often stop taking insulin, even if they have been taking more than 100 units a day.

Furthermore, some people with little or no need for insulin may in fact have many more serious medical complications than those who take insulin. Serious vascular complications can occur with only mild blood sugar elevations, even with good control, whether or not a person takes insulin. The severity of the overall diabetes condition cannot be correlated solely to whether the person takes insulin or how much he takes.

June and Barbara: Is it possible for non-insulin-dependent diabetics to turn into insulin-dependent diabetics?

Dr. Lodewick: More than 80% of people with diabetes do not require insulin. They can get control without insulin *if* they can lose weight, follow a diet and exercise program, and get their blood sugar back to normal (60 to 120 mg/dl). The problem is that people can feel well with high blood sugars—even as high as 300 mg/dl! Such people tend to ignore diabetes, thinking that it's causing them no problems. Unfortunately not only can it be causing problems, diabetes researchers have found that such high blood sugars can also cause accelerated aging as well as diabetes complications. It is also thought by some—myself included—that the longer the blood sugar stays high, the greater the chances are that people with Type II diabetes will eventually wear down their own insulin-producing beta cells and develop Type I (insulin-dependent) diabetes. Therefore, if you are a non-insulin-dependent diabetic, you should attempt to keep your blood sugars normal to avoid the possible eventual need for insulin.

June and Barbara: We sometimes find that older men are particularly resistant to taking insulin, either because it frightens them or they figure that there's no point in doing so at their age. Do you have ways of convincing older men to take insulin when it's required for their diabetes control?

Dr. Lodewick: It depends on whether they indeed have Type I (insulin-dependent) diabetes and on how much longer they want to live. Some older men who've never been ill are shocked (as are younger people) that they should be the victim of such a potentially debilitating disease. Unless and until they get over the shock, they will never admit that diabetes is a problem for them and will refuse insulin. To insist that such a man must take insulin is a mistake. It will cause him to have only anger and distrust. In this case, it's probably better to let him linger on in the hope that he doesn't have diabetes, even though he does. Then, during the course of treatment, the doctor can point out that his blood sugars are high and that this may cause him to "slow down" or that some of the slowing down he seems to be experiencing is a result of high blood sugar. Finally, it may sink in that insulin (which today is not that difficult or painful to administer) may help to prevent him from slowing down so that he can continue to have a meaningful and productive life for all of his allotted years.

June and Barbara: We have also met many younger and middle-aged men who are tough as horseshoe nails and brave as lions in all other aspects of life—military heroes, big rig truck drivers, sky divers, boxers—but who are terrified of sticking needles into themselves. Do you have any experiences with men having this problem, and do you have any ways of helping them overcome their fear?

Dr. Lodewick: It's not uncommon for doctors to see the most masculine of men be the most frightened of needles or the sight of blood. Football players are typically the ones who faint during blood tests or vaccinations, but it can happen to anyone of any age.

A recent case comes immediately to mind. A beautiful, healthy five-year-old boy named Joey suddenly developed signs of diabetes. His blood sugars were in excess of 500 mg/dl. His mom and dad were shocked. They couldn't believe that their wonderful child could have such a terrible affliction as diabetes. They were afraid the he would start having all sorts of problems.

After starting Joey on insulin, I spent considerable time reassuring his mom and dad that everything would be all right. I let them know that he was healthy and would continue to be as long as we could keep his blood sugar reasonably well controlled. Just at that point, I suggested that we do a blood sugar test with a finger stick. Very bravely this youngster put out his finger, and we got a drop of blood for the blood glucose meter reading.

As we were waiting for the result and I was continuing to reassure his mom and dad that everything was fine, I looked over at Joey, who was white as a ghost and passed out cold on his mother's lap. We quickly placed him in a supine position on the floor where he rapidly regained consciousness. Needless to say, his parents were quite alarmed and began to question the validity of all my reassurances. Was passing out another characteristic of diabetes? How many more times was this going to happen? I continued to reassure them but at that moment they weren't prepared to believe me. Fortunately, as time has passed, Joey has done well with no more fainting, and his parents are much more confident about his diabetes therapy.

Besides Joey, I've also seen many grown men faint. In addition, there are many men who are fearful of taking insulin. Some refuse it because the hazard caused by taking insulin (hypoglycemia) may mean the loss of their jobs, especially if the insulin isn't used properly in concert with self-testing of blood sugar (see Chapter 5 on The Working Man). These men will do anything to avoid insulin injections. Many of them are extremely cooperative in following their diet and in using exercise to stave off the need for insulin. To convince them to accept insulin takes quite a bit of bargaining, especially if they feel well at the time. As I keep emphasizing, some people feel reasonably well even with blood sugars in the 300 mg/dl range. These people must be reminded that even though they feel well, rapid aging of the blood vessels may be taking place so that a major medical problem could suddenly emerge. To prevent this aging of the blood vessels, insulin may be necessary.

Sometimes, even if they feel rotten, they will still fight it. Recently, a man walked into my office and recounted a history of a skin condition manifested by boils, yeast and fungus infections, and poor wound healing. Ever since the diagnosis of diabetes, he had never had a blood sugar under 200 mg/dl. Insulin was repeatedly suggested to him and just as repeatedly refused. "I don't want needle marks all over me," was his answer.

He had gone to many doctors, but the skin condition relentlessly continued. He asserted that the doctors didn't know why he had the skin condition and why it wouldn't go away despite medication and meticulous care of the wounds. Although he spent a great deal of money and much time on medical care, he felt increasingly tired and his sex life was rapidly disappearing. His wife was ready to look for another man.

As a last resort, he came to me hoping I could help him in his predicament. I had one simple answer for him: insulin. It would cure all his lingering and progressive problems. He looked at me and finally admitted, "You're right, Doc." With that he reluctantly agreed to it. After starting insulin, he wondered why he'd made such a fuss over it—and, of course, his problems *did* clear up, including those with his wife.

There are other men who will finally recognize the need for insulin but who will only agree to it if someone else—usually their wife or mother—will give it to them. This was the case with one very physically active construction worker I know. By all appearances, you'd have thought he would fear nothing, let alone a meager insulin needle. Others will agree only if they can get the help of some kind of device to aid injection.

June and Barbara: Fortunately, a number of new devices on the market today make it much easier and less painful to inject insulin now than it once was. For example, automatic injectors are easy and inexpensive. You simply fill the syringe, put it into the injector, and then automatically shoot it in so fast you hardly feel it. Actually, when you put the needle in yourself even *without* an automatic injector, it should hardly hurt if you have good injection technique. What these automatic devices do is instantly give you good injection technique. There are now five different automatic injectors available—the Injectomatic from Sherwood Medical, the Autojector and the Diamatic from Ulster Scientific, the Inject-Ease from Palco, and the Instaject II from Jordan Enterprises. With all except the Autojector and the Diamatic, you manually push the plunger to deliver the insulin. With those two, it's automatically delivered.

Another way of cutting down on the emotional trauma of injection is with a new device from Scandinavia called the Insuflon. You insert a thin plastic tube into your abdominal area, and then for five days you can inject your insulin through its resealable opening. It's true that you have to insert the plastic tube with a needle (which you then remove), but that's the only time you have to stick a needle into yourself for five days, no matter how many shots you take a day. June has used the Insuflon and finds she is not aware of it even when she is skiing or bike riding. You can also take showers or baths with no problem. The Insuflon wouldn't even show under a man's swimsuit. One small problem is that some people report getting mild skin irritation in the area where the adhesive foam pad is attached. Unfortunately, the manufacturer recommends treating this condition with a hydrocortisone cream, which in certain people can elevate the blood sugar.

Another way out for needlephobes is a jet injector, which does not use needles at all. The insulin is delivered in a thin stream literally as fast as a jet flies. In effect, the insulin itself becomes the needle. Most people report that jets, if used properly, are as painless as flicking your index finger against yourself. The bad news about jet injectors is the cost—they can run as high as $800. The good news is that using a jet injector may improve your diabetes control because the insulin is absorbed faster and better since it doesn't pool at the injection site the way it sometimes does with needles. Have any of your patients had good—or not so good—experiences with using jet injectors?

Dr. Lodewick: Yes, a good many of my patients have used jet injectors. Actually I was introduced to them by the same RCA engineer, Ed, whom I mentioned earlier. Engineers are always looking for perfection. This engineer was looking for perfection in blood sugars without having to make so many needle injections. His solution was the Medi-Jector. This allowed him to give himself insulin before each meal and at bedtime—four times a day—without having to use the needle. This got him close to the perfection that engineers seek.

An even more gratifying case was a 15-year-old diabetic boy. He came to me because he was thin and short and wanted my opinion as to whether diabetes was affecting his growth and development—and what he could do about it if it was. He weighed only 99 pounds and was just over five feet tall. I discovered he was taking only one shot of insulin in the morning. A random blood sugar test taken during his office visit showed levels over 500 mg/dl. There was no doubt that his poor diabetes control was having an adverse effect on his growth and development. My suggestion was that to get better control, he had to work with both his diet and with more insulin. A minimum of two injections a day and preferably three would certainly help. There was one problem: this young man had a psychological aversion to insulin needles. Although he was a brilliant straight-A student who clearly understood the advantage of taking two or three doses, he hated the needle and refused to subject himself to it more than once a day. The Medi-Jector was the answer to this dilemma. His control improved remarkably, and in less than a year he gained 30 pounds and three inches in height.

Parents of young diabetic children also find it easier to use one of the jet injectors on them rather than sticking them with a needle.

But before jumping on the bandwagon or making the decision to use a jet injector, there are some disadvantages to consider. You already mentioned the high price—although this cost may be made up by the savings of not having to buy syringes, and some insurance companies do cover jet injectors. They also have to be cleaned and sterilized every two weeks, a process that can take about a half hour. But probably the main disadvantage of jet injectors is their bulkiness. It's much easier to use a Novolin Pen (a dial-a-dose insulin delivery pen) or to carry a syringe than to lug around a jet injector, especially for someone on the move. It's not an uncommon experience of many who purchase jet injectors that they go back to using syringes within six months.

June and Barbara: Another way of delivering insulin without needles (in a sense) is the insulin pump. Many men have read advertisements for insulin pumps and are curious about how they work and whether they are the ideal solution for all Type I diabetics. We're aware that some physicians favor them and recommend them to many of their patients, while others shy away from them for one reason or another. Where do you stand on pumps?

Dr. Lodewick: Pumps are the premier example of what I call the *basal–bolus system*. To understand what this means, you have to first understand the workings of the normal pancreatic beta cells, which the insulin pumps have been designed to emulate. (Pumps are sometimes referred to as artificial beta cells.) Normal beta cells are constantly secreting a small amount of insulin, even during prolonged periods of not eating (fasting or starvation). This constant secretion is referred to as the *basal insulin*. Larger amounts of insulin are secreted in response to food or when your blood sugar rises for some other reason. This is called the *bolus insulin*.

The basal insulin is crucial in preventing the accelerated breakdown of body proteins and fat that will occur without it. In fact, it's because insulin-dependent diabetics lack this basal insulin that they are prone to ketoacidosis, which we previously discussed at length. This is a very important concept to understand, because if the insulin pump malfunctions and insulin isn't replaced by added manual injections, ketoacidosis may occur. This explains why if you have insulin-dependent diabetes, you must continue to take at least a basal amount of insulin, even when you're sick with vomiting. You may even need extra insulin to offset the increased demand during periods of stress or illness. What you may fear is that if you don't eat and continue to take insulin, you may get hypoglycemia. Generally in illness this doesn't happen. What is also important to understand is that even in the presence of basal insulin, hypoglycemia will not occur because the counterregulatory hormones of adrenaline, glucagon, and cortisol are working against that basal insulin to keep your blood sugar high enough for the proper functioning of your brain and other tissues, even when food isn't available.

The present insulin pumps have been designed to inject this basal dose automatically just under the skin in the abdominal area in the same places where syringe-injected insulin would go. They deliver the basal insulin as a steady amount of regular insulin every few seconds at a basal rate generally between 0.4 and 2.0 units per hour.

In addition to the basal insulin, the pumps can also (by the press of a button) deliver additional regular insulin (the only kind used in pumps) before meals or snacks. This is the bolus insulin. It's designed to copy a normal pancreas's rapid secretion of insulin in response to food or rising blood sugar. The amount of bolus insulin that is given can be anywhere between 1.0 and 12 units, depending on such factors as time of day, your actual blood sugar level prior to the meal, and what you're going to eat. The bolus should be given anywhere between 10 and 60 minutes prior to eating. Each person using a pump has differing basal and bolus insulin requirements. It's a very individual thing. The amount of basal and bolus insulin is strictly determined by an estimate based on the amount of carbohydrate you'll be eating and the amount of exercise you plan to do, with the help of five to seven blood sugar tests per day.

There's been a great deal of controversy over the use of pumps. They were first tested in the research setting to make sure they worked perfectly and to iron out all possible complications and side effects before they were used by the general public. For many people, blood sugar control has been far better with pumps than that obtainable using one to four injections per day. In my own practice, patients have come to me with "brittle" (unstable) diabetes, unable to succeed in obtaining good blood sugar control. Their blood sugars have fluctuated markedly from very high (over 400 mg/dl) to very low (under 40 mg/dl) for no discernible reason with only minimal changes in food, insulin dose, or physical activity. Thanks to the insulin pump, I have seen patients such as these gain control that they were never before able to achieve, some having tried hard for 20 years or more. The following case describes such a situation.

PUMP SUCCESS STORY

Tom had struggled with diabetes control for years, but was never able to get a negative urine test for sugar without having an insulin reaction. He went all over the country seeking help: to the Joslin Clinic in Boston, to the Pritikin Program in Southern California, and to numerous doctors in the Northeast before coming to me. After seeing him and finding many complications, I concluded that better control would help. Since none of the great specialists he had seen had been able to help him get good control, I suggested an insulin pump. With that he gained the control he had never had before. Now most of his urine tests were negative without insulin reactions, and his glycohemoglobin level dropped to 8 to 9% from well over 12%.

Unfortunately, this success story has an unhappy ending. Tom went on to develop continuing medical problems. It has since been brought out by medical researchers that once certain diabetes complications advance significantly, good control may not prevent or slow down their progress. That's why I feel it's so important to get good control *before* complications develop.

June and Barbara: It is exciting to see how well Tom's diabetes control responded to the use of the pump; this might motivate other men to want to use one. We might even ask, why don't all insulin-dependent people use a pump?

Dr. Lodewick: The enthusiasm that you see initially in patients who tried pumps in the early 1980s has been dampened by some of the drawbacks to their use.

1. They are not what you'd call a natural addition to the sensual human body and are not, therefore, very attractive to wear. This was particularly true of the earlier models. Now they are reasonably small and can be worn like a beeper or on a belt or holster concealed in the pouch of a garment. Still some people don't like to have them around.

2. The site of injections is subcutaneous and a long catheter is needed to carry the insulin from the pump to the injection site, which must be kept sterile.

The needle or Sof-set should be changed every two or three days. Infection is a possible side effect in certain susceptible people no matter how carefully the needle is inserted or how sterile it is.

3. Most of the pumps are not waterproof, so they are not wearable in a Jacuzzi or during water sports.

4. For more freedom, pumps sometimes have to be detached during times of sexual activity so they don't get in the way of lovemaking.

5. A possible medical problem with the pump is the rapid development of ketoacidosis if the insulin supply is cut off due to a clog or breakdown in the pump or a leak in the catheter. Remember, if the pump stops working or the catheter leaks, the pump user is getting no insulin, and without insulin, especially in a very brittle person, ketoacidosis can occur quickly.

June and Barbara: Considering all the pluses and minuses, which men would you counsel to try a pump?

Dr. Lodewick: Let's first consider those for whom an insulin pump may not be appropriate. Since it hasn't been scientifically documented that perfect control (which is the ideal reason for using a pump) does any better than fair to good control over a 16-year period, then this would eliminate elderly diabetics. An 80-year-old's interests would not include the use of a pump, at least not in their present stage of development. Then there are those who use alcohol or drugs, for which poor judgment might result in improper use of the pump. People who are not cooperative in frequent blood sugar testing or who do blood sugar testing improperly would not be appropriate candidates, either. Since the use of an insulin pump needs considerable understanding both of the amount of insulin that the pump should deliver and the actual mechanics of the pump and what to do in case of malfunction, it wouldn't be appropriate for a person who doesn't have 24-hour access to a physician or professional person familiar with its use.

Some physicians do not recommend a pump when a person already has serious complications because once the complications have gone that far, they can't be reversed even if good control can be achieved. So why put such a person through the hassle of using a pump? My experience is different. In my judgment many complications *can* be reversed, and improved control might prevent further complications from developing. I've also seen eye and kidney complications stabilized after good control has been established.

Finally, if good control can be obtained with diet, exercise, and two to four insulin injections a day, as it can in many people, then there would be little expectation for improved control with the pump. Such people would not be pump candidates.

June and Barbara: In spite of these negative aspects you point out, we find there are many diabetics on the West Coast who happily wear pumps. Two of our SugarFree Center managers (in Del Mar and Torrance, California) are on late model pumps with very successful results. The new MiniMed Sof-set eliminates the problem of having a needle inserted in you all the time, allowing more diabetics to find pump wearing comfortable. There are even Pumper Clubs in Southern California where wearers get together and exchange ideas. Based on your own experience with patients, which ones have had the greatest success with pumps?

Dr. Lodewick: Here's my list of good pump candidates:

1. Those who want it no matter what the costs or the difficulties with use, even if they have good control without it.

2. Youths—the younger the onset of diabetes, the greater the chance that good control may prevent complications.

3. Those who have failed to get good control despite their hardest efforts, including multiple doses of insulin, good diet, and frequent blood sugar testing.

4. Women who are considering pregnancy.

June and Barbara: Did you ever wear a pump yourself?

Dr. Lodewick: Yes, I did. In fact, I had a strange question put to me while I was wearing it. One of my women patients gasped when she saw it and said, "Gee, you really have a serious case, don't you?" This indicated a total lack of understanding of diabetes. I thought I had educated this woman properly, but evidently not. I had to explain that a pump is just another way of delivering insulin and a way to get better control.

I did get better control while I was using the pump, but it was too much of an annoyance for me to continue using it. This was before the advent of the Sof-set, so the needle was always in my belly; it hurt and it caused big black and blue areas (hematomas), especially if the needle moved in and out with exercise. Worse yet, I didn't find it conducive to my sex life! Other than that, it was fine. I've since gone back to taking multiple injections of insulin with the help of the Novopen, and I get almost as good control, occasionally better, if I am especially careful with my diet.

June and Barbara: We know many diabetics, including June, who've had a lot of success with what's called "the poor man's pump." This is your basal–bolus system, only without using the actual pump. You take a very long range insulin dose (for example, Ultralente) once or twice a day to provide the basal dose and then you bolus with regular insulin before each meal. This can be done by injecting with needles. June, however, has a unique way of doing it, which you couldn't call a "poor man's" method since she shoots her basal dose with a Medi-Jector and her bolus dose with an Insuflon.

But no matter how you take it, one of the great fears of those who take insulin is that their blood sugar will suddenly drop very low (called hypoglycemia, insulin shock, or insulin reaction) and they will embarrass themselves in front of their friends or colleagues. Our friend, author, and diabetes specialist Dr. Richard K. Bernstein once quit his job during an insulin reaction (fortunately, he got it back). Insulin reactions can also be dangerous in certain circumstances. Yet there are ways to prevent them. Can you give us some background information on insulin reactions and your suggestions for coping with them?

Dr. Lodewick: First, we have to face the fact that insulin reactions can occur in anyone who uses insulin. I must admit that I've suffered more than one. It's important to realize, however, that most insulin reactions are avoidable. There is no reason to have repeated hypoglycemic attacks and need to be taken off to the emergency room several times a year, as I've seen in a few cases.

Reactions generally occur when blood sugar levels drop below 50 mg/dl. Normal blood sugar is generally between 60 and 120 mg/dl. This means that there is only about 1 teaspoon of sugar (5 grams) in your bloodstream at any one time. This is quite remarkable since the average person may barrage his or her digestive system with 15 to 60 teaspoons of sugar per day. (The average diet contains 75 to 300 grams of simple or complex carbohydrate, most of which is converted to sugar in the body.) Thus, it's easy to see that if you're a well-controlled diabetic you could easily develop an insulin reaction by merely omitting as little as one fruit or starch/bread exchange, which contains an equivalent of 3 teaspoons of sugar. A biochemist patient of mine proved this when he skipped two starch/bread exchanges and found his blood sugar down to nearly 30 mg/dl several hours later.

For the nondiabetic, the pancreas secretes into the bloodstream only the amount of insulin that's necessary to keep the blood sugar level at one teaspoon (60 to 120 mg/dl). In contrast, since Type I diabetics must inject insulin, the blood insulin level depends more upon the amount of insulin and/or the speed with which it is absorbed from the injection site. For instance, it's absorbed more slowly from your leg than from your arm or belly. This may explain some of the erratic control that you may have noticed.

Another factor you must consider is that your insulin requirements can drop by one-third or more if you add exercise to your daily program. The biochemist I previously mentioned also had a problem with the effects of lowering blood sugar from exercise. One holiday season he played three hours of basketball with his family, which was much more exercise than he was accustomed to. He had no problem on the day of playing basketball, but the next day he passed out from low blood sugar. From this experience, he learned that the effect from exercise can be extended for up to 24 hours after the period of exercise. Up to five teaspoons of sugar or the equivalent may be needed per hour during the period of exercise, as well as extra calories or a reduction in insulin before and after exercise.

So we can summarize by saying that most reactions are caused by too much insulin, insufficient food, too much exercise, or a combination of these.

June and Barbara: We've found that many Type I's are taught how to inject themselves with insulin, but they are given little information about recognizing reactions and handling them. We're certain you will agree with us that this is a potentially hazardous situation and that you can't learn too much about it if you want to stay out of trouble and, equally important, not cause trouble for others.

Dr. Lodewick: Yes, recognizing a low blood sugar reaction is extremely important so that proper treatment can be given. One of the most striking features of a reaction is the speed with which it comes on. You can be feeling perfectly fine when all of a sudden you get shaky, nervous, sweaty, anxious, irritable, and hungry. There may be other telltale signs such as the sensation of a rapid heartbeat or numbness of the lips. These symptoms are generally attributed to overproduction of adrenaline in response to the low blood sugar. If you don't eat or drink something to bring it up, blood sugar will continue to drop into the range of 20 to 40 mg/dl, which is not enough sugar to supply the brain. When there's a lack of sugar to the brain, the result is similar to a lack of oxygen to the brain. A whole variety of symptoms can occur and each individual may manifest different ones. You may get sleepy or cantankerous, you may cry, complain of blurred vision, be nauseous, or get a headache. You may develop strange behavior: anger, delirium, confusion, and even go so far as to lose consciousness or have a seizure.

Many of these symptoms aren't harmful to you, but in certain situations they can become dangerous. In my practice I've seen many bad insulin reactions cause serious automobile accidents. I've come to the conclusion that people who can't prevent severe insulin reactions despite their best efforts shouldn't drive. Fortunately, few people fall into this category. Most of you can avoid a reaction if you simply take a blood sugar test before driving. Your blood sugar should be over 100 mg/dl. You should always keep glucose tablets in the car, as well as blood sugar testing apparatus in case you're caught in stalled traffic. I cannot emphasize this too much.

I must also point out that it's often easy to fail to notice warning symptoms of hypoglycemia. You may overlook them when exercising heavily since some of the symptoms of low blood sugar are the same as the normal effects of exercise and competition (for example, sweating and nervousness). When you are in deep concentration on some task you may slip into hypoglycemia without noticing it. In addition, there are some diabetics who, for various reasons, do not get the typical hypoglycemic warning symptoms. Others, as years go by, either become unaware of their warning symptoms or the symptoms become less evident until extreme sleepiness, confusion, or loss of consciousness occurs. These people need to take more frequent blood sugar tests, and they dare not drive without testing first. They also should discuss with their doctors what they can do to avoid hypoglycemic reactions.

June and Barbara: What do you suggest men should eat when they have a reaction?

Dr. Lodewick: This, fortunately, is pretty clear-cut, but some diabetics make it tricky. Some like to have a mild insulin reaction because they think it gives them the chance to eat something sweet such as their favorite candy—a Milky Way or Snickers bar. What must be remembered, though, is that all it may take to raise your blood sugar from 30 to 80 mg/dl is less than two teaspoons of sugar or the equivalent. Any more than that, such as a whole Milky Way, may raise it to 300 to 400 mg/dl. However, since extreme hunger is a common symptom of low blood sugar, it's not unusual for a hypoglycemic diabetic to eat everything that's in front of him—even the entire contents of the refrigerator!

For mild insulin reactions you can get the equivalent of two teaspoons of sugar from any of the following: two to four glucose tablets (Dextrosols, DextroTabs, or B-D Glucose Tablets), four ounces of orange juice or Coca-Cola, seven or eight Life-Savers, one tablespoon of honey, or two tablespoons of raisins. It is probably reasonable for you to eat a little more, even if it does make your blood sugar go higher than normal. In that way you can alleviate your symptoms more quickly and make certain that your blood sugar doesn't continue to drop, especially if you've mistakenly taken too much insulin or skipped part of a meal. This will prevent your thinking processes from being affected, particularly if the circumstances require a quick-thinking brain. If your blood sugar *does* go too high, cutting back slightly on the upcoming meal should help you get it back on keel.

As I mentioned, many diabetics, as they descend from alertness to confusion, don't recognize that they are having an insulin reaction. If you are one of these, you must alert those around you—family, colleagues at work, friends—to be on the lookout for evidence of hypoglycemia. Warn them that you may stubbornly refuse to believe that your blood sugar is low and may refuse treatment, but that they must *insist*. Make sure they know what to give you. If you argue with them about taking the treatment, tell them to make you test your blood sugar—if you're still capable of doing it.

At home and at your workplace, as well as in your automobile glove compartment, golf bag, tennis bag, or the like, keep some Insta-Glucose, Glutose, or Insulin Reaction Gel. These are gels that can be squeezed into your mouth where they are absorbed, even if you're too far gone to chew. Let your companions know about these treatments for hypoglycemia and show them where you keep them.

Caution them, however, to never put anything into your mouth if you become unconscious or are convulsing. This could choke you. At this point you need an injection of Glucagon (Eli Lilly produces an emergency kit available by prescription). Make sure your family members and close friends know how to administer it (see Appendix E for procedure). After the Glucagon brings you around, you should eat more upon awakening (usually within 15 minutes). Then your doctor should be notified about what happened. The only other solution if you are unconscious is for the paramedics to be called—a costly and disrupting experience.

A special word about hypoglycemia for Type II men on oral diabetes medications. In general, hypoglycemia is less risky for you. It's most likely to occur if you have just started on oral medicines or if you're sick and not eating well and continue to take your medication. When people with Type II diabetes have nausea or poor appetite, I generally recommend holding off on diabetes medicines unless you know your blood sugar is high.

June and Barbara: We wonder if you've had Type I diabetics tell you that they can always tell by how they feel whether their blood sugar is high or low. June finds this very difficult to believe, as she readily confesses that she usually hasn't the slightest idea what her blood sugar is without using a meter to test it. She's so dubious of her own judgment that she won't even eat something when she feels low (and hungry!) unless she tests to verify that it's the real thing and not just her imagination. Maybe we should even ask, do you yourself recognize your highs and lows easily?

Dr. Lodewick: My own experience is that I often have the very same symptoms when low or high, and I can't tell which it is without testing. For instance, on one occasion when I was feeling sleepy and thirsty, I assumed my blood sugar was high. But when I tested it, I found it was actually low. On another occasion, with identical symptoms, it was high instead. Only blood sugar testing can clear up this confusion.

But like you, I've heard some diabetics emphatically insist that they can tell what their blood sugars are by how they feel. They're so certain that they don't do blood sugar testing to find out. Some probably think they know the state of their blood sugar because they drank too much beer or ate too much food and have a good hunch what the result of that kind of activity is. But studies have shown that different people have different reactions to a given blood sugar level. Some feel miserable at normal levels and great at 250 mg/dl—or great at normal levels and miserable at 250 mg/dl. Also, there are other conditions that can cause the same symptoms, and you may be fooled into assuming blood sugar is responsible when it's actually heart palpitations, cardiac arrhythmias, thyroid disorders, anxiety, or something similar. These other conditions need to be identified so that proper treatment can be given in cases when blood sugar tests normal but symptoms of low or high blood sugar are present. So don't rely on your feelings; rely on your meter.

June and Barbara: It's often said that among Type I diabetics, reactions are the price you have to pay for "tight control." Could you give us a definition of tight control so men will know what they're buying at that price?

Dr. Lodewick: By tight control, we mean trying to keep blood sugars virtually normal at all times. This is very difficult to do under most circumstances, particularly for Type I diabetics. To help you achieve tight control, your physician may suggest several insulin doses per day or even have you try an insulin pump. In the hospital under the careful scrutiny of nurses, dietitians, and laboratory technicians, you're given instructions on the use of insulin, insulin pump operation and care, and blood sugar–insulin algorithms (rules that tell you what your dose should be based on your current blood sugar). These instructions help you to adjust your insulin dose to get as good control as possible without provoking low blood sugar reactions. If tight diabetes control can't be obtained in the hospital, where there is close supervision, it's unlikely that it can be done on an outpatient basis. If it *can* be obtained in the hospital, then it's possible outside the hospital, too.

June and Barbara: There's always a tendency for diabetics to blame every physical problem they have on diabetes. In many cases, it isn't necessarily so. To clear up the confusion on this point, can you enumerate which male (and unisex) problems, conditions, and diseases can actually be brought on or exacerbated by diabetes?

Dr. Lodewick: As Dr. Jovanovic-Peterson indicated in *The Diabetic Woman*, diabetes can certainly aggravate a number of underlying problems, especially if the diabetes is out of control. These include skin infections, boils and abscesses, and fungal or yeast infections of the skin, nails, and mucous membrane (mouth and penis), all of which are less likely to develop in well-controlled diabetes. Other problems are gum and dental disease, high blood fats (cholesterol) and triglycerides (which may return to normal with good control), heart and vascular disease, hypertension, depression, headaches, exhaustion, fatigue, and lack of motivation to do anything.

On the other hand, just because a person has diabetes does not mean that all physical problems are caused by it. A young woman I knew with diabetes was unable to have a child. This was attributed to her diabetes. When she sought my attention, I discovered that she coincidentally had hypothyroidism, which was not caused by her diabetes. I was happy to help her become pregnant. Before you get the wrong idea, I did this by prescribing thyroid replacement, which restored her fertile state. She went on to have two beautiful children.

I've seen a number of other medical disorders including skin disease (acne), heart rhythm disorders requiring pacemakers, congenital heart valve disorders, hypertension, gallbladder and liver disease, and other glandular conditions that also had been erroneously diagnosed as diabetes-related problems. Because of the misdiagnosis, the patients had not been properly cared for. So when you have unusual symptoms, don't always attribute them to diabetes. Make sure there isn't some other reason. Check with your doctor.

June and Barbara: Damage to the eyes is one of the most common complications of diabetes. Let's take up the important subject of how to prevent it. Since it's even treatable by laser therapy if diagnosed early, tell us how often a diabetic man should have an eye check-up.

Dr. Lodewick: *Diabetic retinopathy*, the disease of the area in the back of the eye responsible for vision, has been the number one cause of blindness in the United States, Great Britain, Europe, and Scandinavia since 1974. There are a number of reasons postulated as to why vision is lost in diabetes, but high on the list is poor control. A 1990 study reported in the *New England Journal of Medicine* substantiated this. Glycohemoglobin levels were used to determine the degree of control. Severe retinopathy developed in only 2.9% of patients with glycohemoglobin levels below 8.4%, in 12.5% of those with glycohemoglobin levels between 8.4 and 9.0%, and in 44% of those with glycohemoglobin levels over 9.9%. These figures speak for themselves. If you aren't already in good control, work with your doctor, your diet, your exercise, and your medicine until you get your glycohemoglobin below 8.4%, if at all possible.

The hidden danger is that severe diabetic retinopathy can occur without your knowing it, and you may not find out until too late to prevent vision loss. Two major research studies (the Diabetic Retinopathy Study and the Early Treatment of Diabetic Retinopathy Study) have shown that vision loss caused by diabetic retinopathy can be prevented if laser treatment is done early enough. This is why it is so important to make sure that your retinas (the area of the eye responsible for vision) are being checked regularly by an ophthalmologist trained in diabetic retinopathy.

The American College of Ophthalmology has developed guidelines that identify characteristics of quality eye care. They suggest eye examinations be done according to the following schedule:

Recommended Eye Examination Schedule for People with Diabetes

Diabetic Category	*Frequency of Eye Check-Up*
Child	At age 13, then yearly or more depending on presence of retinopathy
Adult	Yearly
Adult with retinopathy	Every 4 to 6 months
Adult with hypertension	At diagnosis, then yearly
Adult with sudden vision loss	Immediately, unless physician can explain it by fluctuating blood sugar
Adult on medicine for other serious health problems	Soon after beginning

Also, to check your own vision periodically and to make sure your entire retinal area is seeing 100%, you can use the Amsler Grid (see Appendix F). Follow the directions carefully. If all the lines are not straight and all the squares not the same size, check with your doctor or ophthalmologist right away.

June and Barbara: Since an estimated 40 to 50% of people with diabetes also have high blood pressure (hypertension), could you provide some instruction on how to attend to that problem when a man faces both of these risks?

Dr. Lodewick: In hypertension the risk of heart attack or stroke progressively increases as the systolic blood pressure increases. With diabetes, that risk is much greater. The problem is how and when to treat the blood pressure. Some research studies indicate that if hypertension can be effectively treated or prevented, this will prevent the progression of kidney failure that is seen in so many patients with diabetes. The strength of these studies is so good that there is some speculation that blood pressure medication should be tried in diabetics even before it would otherwise be used in nondiabetics.

Generally, most physicians do not prescribe blood pressure medication unless all nonpharmacological methods (including restricted salt use, diet modification, and exercise) have failed and blood pressure is above 140/90 mmHg. (Blood pressure is the force of the blood on the walls of the arteries as measured in millimeters of mercury, abbreviated mmHg.) Some ongoing studies are documenting whether medications will prevent the development of hypertension and/or kidney disease in diabetics, even when the diabetics have normal blood pressure when beginning the medication.

Even before knowing the results of these studies, most experts think that control of blood pressure will help prevent coronary heart disease in diabetics because there would only be one risk factor (diabetes) for heart disease instead of two (diabetes and hypertension). So if six to ten weeks of effort to control blood pressure with weight loss, exercise, and calorie and sodium restriction fail to get blood pressure below 140/90 mmHg, medication should definitely be considered. However, it is important to make sure that the medication is free of significant side effects.

Until the mid-1980s, diuretics and beta blockers were considered to be the prime antihypertensive medicines. The diuretics include thiazides, Hygroton, Hydrodiuril, and Lasix; the beta blockers are Inderal, Tenormin, and Lopressor. Unfortunately for people with diabetes, these medications have significant side effects that can easily nullify any good effect they have on lowering blood pressure. These side effects include raising blood sugar, raising total cholesterol while lowering the beneficial HDL cholesterol, and dangerously lowering mineral levels such as potassium.

Fortunately, since the mid-1980s, a number of newer antihypertensive medications have become available that have little effect, or even a beneficial effect, on lipids, potassium, and insulin levels. Some of these include ACE inhibitors such as captopril, enalopril, and prinivil; calcium channel blockers such as diltiazem, Procardia, and verapamil; and alpha-1 blockers such as doxazosin, prazosin, and terazosin. The hope is that one or more of these will be more helpful in lowering the mortality rate caused by uncontrolled hypertension.

June and Barbara: Diabetics are likely to have higher levels of cholesterol and blood fats than nondiabetics. We've even read that high blood sugar may cause elevation of LDLs (low-density lipoproteins, or "bad" cholesterol) and lowering of HDLs (high-density lipoproteins, or "good" cholesterol). What is your advice to diabetic men on the cholesterol problem?

Dr. Lodewick: Cholesterol screening is definitely a must for diabetic men because arteriosclerotic, vascular, and heart diseases, in which blood fats play a role, are so prevalent with diabetes. While such vascular and heart disease is developing, however, there are frequently no symptoms. So high blood cholesterol can be present 20 to 30 years or more before it finally becomes manifest as a heart attack or stroke. This was vividly brought home to me just a few months ago.

HIGH CHOLESTEROL PLUS DIABETES EQUALS HEART ATTACK RISK

One of my patients, Dan, only 36 years of age and presumably healthy, came in for his annual physical. Diabetic since age 15, he had no health problems, ran a successful company, and played heavy basketball for two hours at a time several times a week. His only asymptomatic problem was a high blood cholesterol level for which he refused to take medicine.

Since he had no symptoms of heart problems, I questioned myself on whether I should spend his money getting an electrocardiogram. As it turned out, I was glad I had him do it, although the test was normal. Two weeks later he called to say that he'd had "indigestion" the night before and his co-workers suggested that he call me to discuss it. When I recommended another electrocardiogram, he protested, insisting that he'd just had a normal one. At my insistence that it could be something serious, he reluctantly agreed to come in right away.

Sure enough, the test showed evidence of a myocardial infarction (heart attack). Subsequently, he underwent a triple coronary artery bypass, which I'm glad to say was successful. He's now back to his usual energetic lifestyle.

Dan had a dual problem—diabetes and high blood cholesterol. When both these conditions exist, both have to be attended to. People with diabetes have an accelerated incidence of heart disease when their cholesterol is high. If at all possible, you should keep your total cholesterol under 200, your "bad" LDL cholesterol under 130, and your "good" HDL cholesterol over 40.

June and Barbara: You ordered an electrocardiogram on Dan although he was only 36. How often should this test be done?

Dr. Lodewick: I think it's important for every man to have a baseline electrocardiogram to make sure it's normal even at a young age. Then it can be repeated at varying intervals of every one to four or five years depending on how he's doing.

In some circumstances, a stress electrocardiogram is also advisable. This is an electrocardiogram done with exercise to stress the heart to see if it causes changes in the electrocardiogram that might indicate underlying heart disease. A cost of $150 to $250 is a fair amount of expense to have to put out for such a test, but in a case such as Dan's it might show possible anginal heart disease (heart disease caused by poor circulation to the heart which causes chest pain and heart attacks) before a heart attack actually occurs. I have seen many men in whom a stress electrocardiogram was positive for heart disease even though they didn't have any symptoms. It was important to know about this since they could be treated with medicine or even surgery to prevent a heart attack, or at least they could be cautioned to avoid excessive stress and heavy exercise (such as snow shoveling or basketball) that might induce a heart attack. I think that all men with diabetes, high cholesterol, and a family history of heart disease should have a stress electrocardiogram every four to five years.

June and Barbara: From this, it's clear that cholesterol testing and control are good preventive medicine for diabetic men. When they do have the test, what are the cholesterol levels they should aim for?

Dr. Lodewick: According to the National Institutes of Health (NIH) and the National Education Cholesterol Program, if you are under 30, your cholesterol level should be under 180; if you are over 30, it should be under 200. If you have elevated cholesterol, the risks vary depending on age and cholesterol level, as shown here:

Age	Normal	Moderate Risk	High Risk
20–29	Under 200	Over 200	Over 220
30–39	Under 220	Over 220	Over 240
40+	Under 240	Over 240	Over 260

If your total cholesterol is above normal, then you should also get measurements of your HDL cholesterol and an estimation of your LDL cholesterol and your total blood fats (triglycerides). If your total cholesterol is high but your HDLs are also high and your LDLs are normal, there is less danger, and treatment to lower your cholesterol may not be so important. If, however, your total cholesterol is reasonably good but your HDLs are low, you may be at greater risk, and treatment to raise your HDLs should be considered. The HDL cholesterol averages are shown in the following table. For those in the 25th percentile, this means that only 25% or less of these people have lower HDLs. Therefore, it would be preferable to be in the 75th percentile to cut down on heart risks. In other words, the higher the percentile you are in, the better off you are.

Age	25th Percentile	50th Percentile	75th Percentile
20	39–43	46–51	52–61
20–40	34–38	43–46	49–52
40+	38–41	43–49	51–62

Adapted from *The Lipid Research Clinics Population Studies Data Book*, NIH Publication No. 80, p. 1527, 1980.

POSTSCRIPT

The Ultimate in Delayed Gratification

One of the hallmarks of a winner is the willingness to give up something you want now for something bigger and more important you want in the future. This is what's commonly known as delayed gratification. You've probably had some experience with delayed gratification in your life. Think back to your first car. Unless you had a rich relative bestow one on you, you may have had to work hard and save to buy this big thing you wanted, foregoing a lot of smaller pleasures that would provide instant gratification, such as the latest clothes fads or hamburgers and pizzas and Cokes or movies or rock concerts along the way. After high school graduation, some of your friends may have gone off for a while to enjoy life as surfers or ski bums, but you may have gone to college to prepare yourself for a career or gotten a job to begin the slow climb to a position of responsibility—and financial reward. It's almost certain that you're no stranger to delayed gratification.

Now we're asking you to get even better acquainted with the concept. Diabetes control is the ultimate in delayed gratification. You may spend 5, 10, 20 years or even more denying yourself life's little so-called pleasures—eating and drinking whatever you like whenever you like, kicking back and watching TV instead of taking that run or walk, staying up all night and sleeping until noon on weekends—in short, the immediate gratification of doing what you want whenever you want without thinking about it. And what do you get for giving up this free-wheeling lifestyle? The far-off gratification of not having diabetes complications, a gratification you may not be entirely convinced is important because you are not entirely convinced that complications really await the diabetic profligate. Be convinced. They *do* await you and they're not something you're going to want.

Ron Brown, the medical student we mentioned in the opening of this chapter, was diagnosed diabetic in his early 20s. He looked at his father who was in his 50s. His father was still a young and active man—running an engineering company, skiing, traveling, dining out in interesting restaurants, feeling great, and enjoying himself thoroughly in every way. Without hesitation, Ron decided that he wanted to have that same health, vigor, and enthusiasm for life for all the years that his father was having them. Consequently, he grabbed hold and took control of his diabetes and hasn't let go since. He's in perfect health and is a shoo-in for a lot of years of gratification. The "sacrifices" he's making are small compared to the big rewards he's getting—and will continue to get.

So join Ron and the thousands of other healthy diabetics out there. When the inevitable temptations come your way, control yourself—and your diabetes. By doing so, you will ultimately gain the greatest reward there is—a long lifetime of good health.

The
PSYCHOSOCIAL MAN
• • • •
Meeting the Bear in the Woods

There's a new pop psychology quiz game on the market designed to show how you feel about major life issues such as sex and death, what you think about yourself, and how you would handle challenging situations. For example, try this one.

You're walking through the forest and suddenly a bear looms up in your path. What would you do? Think for a minute or two about how you would handle this emergency. Then read on.

What did you do about the bear? Did you run from it? Did you try to kill it? Did you climb a tree? Hide behind a bush? Stand perfectly still? Or did you do as June, who's a student of Buddhism, did, have a nice talk with the bear? "Hello there, bear. We're both here in the woods together. There's no reason to fight. Let's live in peace and harmony with each other and go on about our business."

What you decided to do about the bear is supposed to indicate how you deal with the problems in your life, perhaps how you deal with your diabetes. Whatever you decided to do, one thing is pretty certain, though. You didn't decide to deny the bear's existence, pretend he wasn't there, and just walk right through him. You knew that if you did, you'd wind up mauled and destroyed.

Diabetes is a bear in every sense of the word. Deny its existence, pretend it isn't there, walk right through it, and you can wind up mauled and destroyed. Unrealistic though this approach may be, it's exactly the approach a number of men take toward diabetes. *Denial* is the key word. If you deny you have diabetes, you can't do anything about dealing with it. When we say denying diabetes, we don't mean not admitting you have it to others. You may freely acknowledge your diabetes to health professionals and family members, even to friends and colleagues. But do you admit it deep down inside yourself or is there still some part of you saying, "This has nothing to do with me"?

They say a person who learns he or she has a chronic disease goes through the four stages Elisabeth Kübler-Ross describes in *On Death and Dying*: denial, anger, depression, and finally, acceptance. Now is the time to work through these stages until you can get to the point with diabetes that June was with the bear: "Hello there, diabetes. We're both here in this body together. There's no reason to fight. Let's live in peace and harmony with each other and go on about our business."

—June and Barbara

W H A T   Y O U ' L L   F I N D   H E R E

DENIAL

DEPRESSION

PANIC ATTACKS

ILLEGAL DRUGS

DEPENDENCY

STRESS

MALE CULTURAL ROLE

MARRIAGE

CHILDREN

June and Barbara: As we mentioned in our Introduction, when we asked in the *Health-O-Gram* for men to write to us with questions that we could answer in this book, we got very few responses. Does this indicate that men have fewer problems? Or are they relying on someone else to take care of their disease? Are they simply ignoring their diabetes or do they remain in deep denial?

Dr. Lodewick: Just as you speculate as to why you got so few questions, I have to speculate as well. For one thing, more women than men may read your *Health-O-Gram*, hoping to pick up new insights. Some men would rather not have to dwell on the subject of diabetes, especially if they feel well and have no problems that they can't get answers to elsewhere, such as reading in-depth books or discussing their problems with their spouse, friends, or doctor. For some, it's part of their masculine nature to hide a defect, which is what they consider diabetes to be. They feel diabetes may provoke pity and they don't want to be pitied. And some men just don't like to burden others with their troubles. So why ask questions? They'd rather take on the burden themselves than bother others with it.

Some men, feeling well with high blood sugars, are not motivated to learn more about their diabetes, not realizing that it can be silently causing problems that won't manifest themselves until the sudden onset of a major complication. So why ask questions? Some, gamblers by nature, rely on the myth of invulnerability and, although acknowledging that complications can occur, are willing to be risk takers and ignore preventive aspects of diabetes management. So, why ask questions?

Finally, many men will deny that diabetes is a problem for them. In one way that's good, because they can avoid the stress of dealing with diabetes. However, it's much worse when it keeps men ignorant of measures that will allow them to live long and productive lives, as little impeded by diabetes as possible.

These are all reasons for men not asking questions, as well as your speculation that some men rely on someone else (for instance, their spouse) to handle the problem of their diabetes.

June and Barbara: Do you find that men more than women tend to keep their diabetes a secret? Perhaps they feel that their careers may be damaged if people are aware of their problem. Also, because men are expected to be strong and invulnerable, do they feel that as a diabetic this image of themselves will be damaged?

Dr. Lodewick: Yes, I do think many men attempt to hide their diabetes. It's not that they necessarily want to keep it a secret, but they are of a more practical nature than women. Their attitude is, what good in the world is it to let other people know that you have diabetes? It will just make them look down on you as inferior or, worse yet, pity you. Who wants that? Men are more likely to have the point of view that "I'd rather discuss from strength than from weakness." In reality, ignorant people who do not know better *do* consider diabetes a weakness.

We all know there are many celebrities and people in show business and great athletes who keep their diabetes a secret for just such reasons. They don't want to jeopardize their careers by exposing their condition to the ignorant and prejudiced segments of the public.

June and Barbara: You're certainly right about that. We know of one very popular woman entertainer who has always been quite open about her diabetes—even appearing in spot announcements for the American Diabetes Association and Juvenile Diabetes Foundation. But her agent once told us that she was trying to soft-pedal her diabetes a bit because she didn't want people who were seeing her in a play or on television to focus on her diabetes rather than on her performance. The ignorant among them might be sitting there open-mouthed waiting to see her topple over at any minute from her "dread disease."

Dr. Lodewick: Then there's the other reason for secrecy that you suggested. Some men fear diabetes will destroy their image of being strong and invulnerable. Still others would be willing to admit that they have diabetes, except that they don't want others to treat them differently, such as a hostess who goes out of her way to prepare them a special meal.

June and Barbara: Depression is thought by some experts to be inner-directed anger. Do you find that men usually express their anger directly—by raging against getting or having diabetes—or do they become depressed over it? Or are these two characteristic stages of a cycle that all people go through with diabetes?

Dr. Lodewick: Depression is a tough subject, as there are so many explanations for it and how it is interwoven with diabetes. Outward anger is one manifestation. If the anger or depression is not controlled and diabetes is neglected, then the man may develop the complications of out-of-control diabetes.

This reminds me immediately of my patient Schmiddy. He was very angered over getting diabetes. He was one giant of a man, strong and energetic. Then diabetes struck him. Treated by a physician whom he initially trusted but who inexplicably let him go as a patient, Schmiddy was enraged by this doctor's seeming indifference. Some men will put complete trust in their doctors and share with them confidential information that they might not even share with their families. Schmiddy was one of these types of individuals. He was therefore understandably upset when this doctor turned him aside. His reaction was to totally ignore his diabetes. He vowed he would never see a doctor again until he was on his deathbed—and only then if he couldn't avoid it.

In the 10 years that followed, all he did was take the same insulin dose that was prescribed by the doctor who had forsaken him. He got his insulin and syringes from friends who were also diabetic. He ate anything he wanted and bragged about his ability to consume a gallon of Take-a-Boost every week (a favorite southern New Jersey sugar-laden drink, similar to Coke syrup). His weight ballooned to over 300 pounds. He worked irregular hours, doing all shifts. Despite all this neglect, he felt well. He was proud of the fact that his decision to ignore his diabetes totally caused him no problems.

Then the roof caved in. He became increasingly irritable, lethargic, and depressed. His feet bothered him. They were cold and felt so burning and numb that he couldn't sleep at night. He had heard about me through his diabetic friends over the years, and he decided to reconsider his vow not to see a doctor again. The time had come.

When he finally sought my attention, he already had major complications. The fatigue and depression were caused by poor control. His glycohemoglobin level was over 12%. (See Chapter 1, The Physical Man, for a discussion of glycohemoglobin.) The burning and numbness were caused by diabetic neuropathy (nerve damage) along with neuritis (inflammation of the nerves). He had lost sensation in his feet to the point where he couldn't feel severely painful stimuli. His blood pressure was high. He had significant eye changes that indicated diabetic retinopathy. His kidneys were spilling protein, showing that he was on his way to diabetic nephropathy (kidney damage). Unfortunately, over the ensuing months, despite his best efforts to take care of himself, he went on to develop severe vision loss, he developed a gangrened toe that had to be amputated, and he had a small stroke.

Schmiddy's case serves to emphasize the importance of preventing complications before they develop. Once complications set in, they may not be reversible. So my advice is not to wait until you are whammed over the head by complications as Schmiddy was, but to do something to prevent them from happening. Don't let anger and depression stand in the way of good diabetes self-care. The good self-care that makes you feel better physically will also make you feel better emotionally and help foster a more optimistic attitude about your future.

Then there are people who are simply susceptible to depression. Although psychiatrist William Glasser, author of *Positive Addiction*, suggests that depression stems from guilt over lack of accomplishment and not achieving what is necessary to gain the praise of others, I'm not so sure of this analysis. There have been some incredibly gifted people who have achieved far beyond the average and yet still have fits of morbid depression. Writers are particularly prone to this problem—for example, Edgar Allan Poe, Charles Dickens, Eugene O'Neill, and more recently, William Styron (who wrote the book *Darkness Visible* about his depression). In my own practice, I've seen many great and kind people who have suffered from this illness. These people must get psychological help, possibly including medication, for their depression; otherwise, not only will they be tortured by their depression, but they will continue to neglect their diabetes.

Unfortunately, some depressed men may refuse the help they need. It is particularly frustrating for family members to see their loved one do harm to himself and yet not be able to persuade him to seek proper help. If this is the case, they should enlist the help of the family physician or clergyman or the man's close friends to encourage him to take the steps necessary to alleviate his depressed state. Anyone who is down on life needs to consider psychological counseling or even the use of antidepressant medication so that the thrill, joy, and meaning of living return to them.

June and Barbara: Another distressing emotion that a diabetic man may experience is panic. A friend of ours who has been diagnosed diabetic for about a year now told us that before he was diagnosed, he had terrible panic attacks that would come upon him suddenly and for no reason. He was exercising regularly and strenuously and eating a fairly healthy diet—not as good as he ate after being diagnosed, but better than most people. He was under some stress at work, but nothing that he hadn't coped with successfully before. Then the mysterious and unpredictable panic attacks began clamping themselves down on him and reducing him to a helpless blob of terror. His doctor sent him to a psychiatrist, but to no avail.

Then, once he was diagnosed diabetic and started taking insulin, the attacks went away, never to return. The doctor didn't seem to relate the attacks to the undiagnosed (and therefore out-of-control) diabetes. Our friend asked us if we'd ever heard of panic attacks related to diabetes, and we had to confess we hadn't.

Not wanting to give up on finding out about this horrifying disorder he had so vividly experienced himself, he continued reading and researching the subject. His efforts were rewarded. Dr. Mark S. Gold in his book, *The Good News About Panic, Anxiety, and Phobias*, tells the tale of a young man who for years experienced panic disorders almost identical to our friend's. During the attacks he had a horrible feeling—as if he were dying. "My heart felt as if it would jump out of my chest. I felt as if I were choking. Then the chills came over me out of nowhere, and the room started spinning. When I tried to get up, I fainted." Even when he wasn't in the throes of panic, he lived in fear that one of these uncontrollable attacks might come on him at the office or, even worse, while driving.

Finally, during a routine physical examination, it was discovered that he had non-insulin-dependent (Type II) diabetes. His panic attacks had been brought on by fluctuations in his blood sugar. In fact, two hours after taking a glucose tolerance test in conjunction with the physical exam, he experienced one of his worst panic attacks.

It struck us that if fluctuations in blood sugar levels can bring on these attacks in undiagnosed diabetics, they could easily do the same in susceptible individuals with diagnosed and out-of-control diabetes. It's hard enough to cope with the demands of caring for a chronic disease without feeling that you're losing your mind on top of it! Dr. Lodewick, have many of your patients experienced these attacks either prior to diagnosis or when their blood sugars were out of control? Did stabilizing their blood sugars take care of the situation or did they also have to have some psychological counseling to bring them around?

Dr. Lodewick: The psychological consequences of uncontrolled diabetes are well known by all physicians who treat diabetes. Depression, lack of concentration, lethargy, and inability to maintain mental acuity or do tasks requiring mental alertness are all observed in out-of-control diabetics. Panic attacks result when a person feels he is not able to cope. Some poorly controlled diabetic men may feel this way, causing them unnecessary—and potentially dangerous—mental anguish. Often when the man normalizes his blood sugar, the panic attacks go away. If they persist, however, the man should seek psychological help, since the attacks may be due to factors other than his diabetes.

I recently treated a man who suffered the exact panic attacks you just described. Jack was a workaholic, married, and the father of a one-year-old and a three-year-old. He was rarely home to enjoy his children and romance his wife. Then he got diabetes and began to be greatly distressed by these panic attacks. He finally sought my attention, wanting to know whether his diabetes was the cause. I recommended blood sugar testing and found that during his attacks, his blood sugar was in the good range of 90 to 140 mg/dl. It was my impression that his panic attacks were not related to blood sugar levels but to the fear that he wouldn't have time in the future to spend with his family because the complications of diabetes would do him in.

After getting psychological and marital counseling, as well as my reassurance that he was not about to collapse with diabetes complications, Jack's panic attacks stopped. He even took two weeks off to enjoy a cruise with his wife.

Although Jack's case was not related to blood sugars, some men do experience an anxious or depressed state when their blood sugars are high. Others have episodes of panic when their blood sugar levels get much below 60 mg/dl. By getting better control and avoiding peaks and valleys in blood sugars, these men do better with their anxieties.

Sometimes men have strange panic-like episodes after taking insulin which defy medical explanation. Their blood sugars are in the good range, but they seem to fear that insulin may cause them problems. After a little education about diabetes and insulin and some reassurance, they usually feel better.

June and Barbara: In spite of the JUST SAY NO campaign, mind-altering drugs continue to be a major temptation in our society. A man who is depressed or angry over his diabetes might be particularly tempted to take drugs because he wants to alter his mind so he can forget about his disease. What are the special hazards of a diabetic man turning to drugs?

Dr. Lodewick: We'll talk about the hazards of the use and abuse of the most popular and widely used drug, alcohol, later in Chapter 3, The Trencherman. But as far as the illicit mind-altering drugs are concerned, I can unequivocally state that their use creates nothing but tragedy. This is definitely what I've witnessed in all the sad cases of destroyed lives and early deaths from drug abuse. Sure, some people have fun with them occasionally and don't get hurt, but why take the chance? And for the diabetic man, the deleterious effects are greatly magnified. Let's consider the drugs group by group.

COCAINE AND CRACK-COCAINE

This is one of the most dangerous drugs on the black market. Take it once and, particularly if you are psychologically susceptible, you may want it again and again, maybe on a monthly, weekly, or even daily basis. Cocaine, although it may give a person delusions of grandeur and omnipotence, can result in loss of appetite and marked weight loss. It can affect judgment, causing you to give yourself incorrect insulin doses. I've seen severe hypoglycemia and convulsions following cocaine use.

Men with diabetes stand a higher risk of heart and vascular complications. Why combine this risk with what researchers in California have learned about cocaine: that it plays a deadly role in heart disease. Studies show that cocaine addicts have daily heart spasms, evident on treadmill testing. These spasms continue for days after withdrawing from cocaine and are aggravated by emotional outbursts, also caused by cocaine. In a Baltimore study of 3000 sudden deaths, 600 were thought to be caused by "cocaine heart attacks."

Cocaine also has an adverse effect on the nervous system. It alters certain blood chemicals called catecholamines. In diabetes these same catecholamines can become depleted. Finally, in autopsies done on six cocaine users who died suddenly (average age 29), it was found that all of them had severe artery disease and blockage. In my own opinion and in the opinion of many who are familiar with cocaine, anyone who uses it, knowing how deadly it is, has to be bordering on insanity. For diabetics, even doubly so!

MORPHINE, HEROIN, MARIJUANA, AND METHADONE

These medicines (and many other analogs of them that are legally or illegally used) can have a multitude of undesirable effects. They may cause higher blood sugars by altering the way sugar is used by the body and possibly by impairing the release of insulin by the beta cells. In addition, they may have a variable effect on the appetite so that blood sugar may be too high or too low. Diabetes control is therefore difficult. Furthermore, if low blood sugar occurs, the drug user may not be able to recognize it himself because of his impaired mental state.

If a diabetic man is using these drugs chronically or is addicted, the following conditions may also result:

increased chance of impotency;

increased possibility of life-threatening infection, aggravated by poor diabetes control; and

increased chance of gangrene and loss of muscle and body weight.

ACID OR LSD

Any man who would use acid, or LSD, knowing it can cause psychosis (inability to see reality) is already out of touch with reality. There is no way diabetes can be managed adequately when a diabetic is on an acid trip. Acid and diabetes in tandem are incompatible with life.

AMPHETAMINE OR SPEED

Amphetamines, or speed, can cause agitation, loss of appetite, and weight loss, while giving you an illusion of power. Convulsions, overdoses of insulin, and death are obvious sequels.

SEDATIVES

Barbiturates and other sedatives, such as sleeping pills, decrease alertness and increase the likelihood of error in good diabetes management.

June and Barbara: That seems to put the lid on drug use. Now let's move to a different topic. All men—as well as all women—have both masculine and feminine aspects to their natures (Yin and Yang). Many men, however, suppress or fail to recognize their feminine side, and this can be detrimental to them. A recent study from Johns Hopkins Medical School showed that among medical school graduates who became doctors and were followed over the years, those who were more in touch with their emotions (for example, who cried relatively easily in emotional situations) had fewer incidences of cancer and heart trouble. Do you have any observations or thoughts on this topic?

Dr. Lodewick: I'm not sure how to respond to this question. Are men allowed to express both the masculine and feminine in their natures? That depends on the society you live in. In the United States many male children learn early on that boys aren't supposed to cry. It's not even considered manly to be sick. Men and boys are pushed to be leaders and providers for their family. They are not encouraged to show weakness or human frailty—these qualities are considered feminine. Men are supposed to be risk takers. In the United States men must have the masculine qualities of leadership, risk taking, strength, and lack of emotional feeling. You see both fathers and mothers looking for these qualities in their sons, but not in their daughters. They may even rear them differently. A little boy is told by mom and dad, "Big boys don't cry," "Don't be a sissy," or "Don't be afraid," whereas a girl is told "Here, mommy will kiss it and make it better."

When boys or men perceive that this is a societal falsehood, they get more in touch with their emotions. They then feel fewer stresses. They may decide they don't have to be the first in everything and to compete with other men and women in fields they're not comfortable, talented, or even interested in. They may drop some of their learned competitive behavior and become more themselves.

Diabetic men, especially, should attempt to accept more of their feminine side and be the best they can be without having to top everyone else. This agrees with what the great physician and diabetologist Elliott Joslin counseled. In my estimation, he had as good insights into what a person with diabetes feels like as any physician I've known, and he didn't even have diabetes. Dr. Joslin advised many men with diabetes to settle for being "second best." This may not be bad advice for anyone. Too many men get unnecessarily depressed if they are not Number 1.

June and Barbara: Dr. Joslin knew whereof he spoke. We heard that his original ambition was to be an obstetrician, but he found that he lacked the manual dexterity to be a really good one. Instead of struggling and stressing himself to become the best in a field in which he would never be more than second best, he switched to diabetes, and the rest is history. Of course, the fact that his mother was diabetic may have contributed to his dedication and success in the field.

Dr. Lodewick: It's true that the realization that you are not suited to a certain field may lead you to discover an area of life in which you can be the best. However, we should get over the idea that you have to be Number 1 in something or you're a failure. Many men can do very good work and contribute to the welfare of their co-workers and their families by being second best. Sometimes they may even choose to allow their wives to run the show and acknowledge a dependency on them. This can be very good for their longevity and possibly for their marriage as well.

For example, when I asked one 87-year-old insulin-dependent diabetic patient of mine how he had lived so long and happily, he answered, "Because of my wife. She babies me." This is most likely a subtle recognition that he depends on her for emotional and inspirational support. He recognizes that dependence, frequently downgraded by some of the more macho elements of our society as feminine, is a characteristic that has stood him in good stead. He likes having a woman behind him.

June and Barbara: While it is often psychologically beneficial for a man to be dependent upon—or mutually dependent with—the woman in his life, sometimes when diabetes is involved it can be carried too far. We often find that women come into the SugarFree Center to learn how to use a blood sugar meter so they can test their husbands or boyfriends who are either "too busy" or simply refuse to take control of their diabetes. In such cases, do you have some techniques to get men to take charge of their diabetes themselves?

Dr. Lodewick: Husbands can be tricky devils. It depends on their nature. Some men send their wives out to look over what's available while they're busy earning the bread. Then, depending on what information their wives come back with (for example, on blood sugar meters), they may decide whether to put the information (or the meters) to good use.

Other men, deceived by the myth of their own invulnerability and feeling reasonably well, will not think it important to visit the doctor or the diabetes center. They figure, why waste the time and the money? Finally, some think that a visit to the doctor or the purchase of a meter is an admission that they have something wrong with them. They look on it as a wound or a chink in their suit of armor. What man wants to admit to his wife or girlfriend that he is not perfect?

Most wives and girlfriends see through this deception. Depending on their ability to make their male counterpart realize that diabetes won't make him less of a man or make them love him less, their man may respond favorably. I know that I felt less of a man when I was first struck by diabetes. Maureen, my wife, made me feel that this wasn't so, which helped me to restore my masculine ego and stir my competitive nature to fight and conquer diabetes.

I also feel that it's impossible for a wife or girlfriend (or anyone else) to take control of a man's diabetes. The man must want to do it himself. Until he decides to take charge himself, no amount of badgering will work.

Some of the techniques I use to help a man take charge include making him realize that diabetes can cause an accelerated aging of the whole body (who wants to get older more quickly?) and making him aware that he can do things to prevent this from happening. I appeal to his competitive nature (which all humans of both sexes have in the sense that they want to be the best they can be), suggesting that he decide on what goals he wants to shoot for: blood sugar control, glycohemoglobin levels, number of calories, exercise plan, and weight. I suggest he get as much knowledge about diabetes as possible so that he'll know what goals are realistically attainable.

June and Barbara: Do you find that diabetic men don't go to the doctor on as regular a basis as diabetic women do? Do they generally wait until something dramatic goes wrong before they come in? If so, can you give us some insights into the male psyche that would explain this? Or do you think that men don't need to go to the doctor as frequently as women do for their diabetes?

Dr. Lodewick: In my own practice, of the last 1000 patients, 512 were women and 488 were men, which is nearly 50–50. I've not been impressed that women have been more regular in coming in for visits than men. In both cases, they come for a thorough physical examination and a medical history report and for the doctor's knowledge to answer questions about the many aspects of diabetes treatment, including consultation on blood sugar testing, weight loss and body-building guidelines, advice on food, insulin adjustment, and just plain encouragement.

Many just come for reassurance that they are doing things right, and some tell me that frequent visits increase their motivation. I have one man who actually asks for more time and more frequent visits. So, if they get this service, I think men are just as likely to come for visits as women.

There are men with diabetes who have come to me and who have not previously seen a physician for many years. Often they are prompted to come only after something dramatic goes wrong. In querying these men, I find almost invariably that they say they got nothing out of their previous visits to their doctor. One case immediately comes to mind.

Lloyd repeatedly urged his family doctor to test him for diabetes because he had a strong family history of it, but because he felt good, his family doctor resisted testing him. When the doctor finally gave in, he discovered Lloyd's blood sugar was over 200 mg/dl. What made things worse was that his family doctor shrugged this off as "a touch of diabetes." Lloyd then had his blood pressure checked by the nurse at his place of work. It was over 200 mmHg. He then sought my help. Even though he felt well, he already had significant retinopathy which needed the attention of a retinal specialist. Indeed, he had much more than a touch of diabetes and had been ignoring the preventive aspects of care because of the cavalier attitude of his doctor.

I think Lloyd is unusual in that he sought out and demanded good care. How many men are not as well educated and would not be as motivated to do the same? I also think that many men, because the core of their lives is to be a good provider, look more at the practical aspect of their medical care. If they feel they are not getting any worthwhile benefits from their physician, they may not see him or her regularly, particularly if it interrupts their work schedule or social engagements.

However, if a physician is thorough, knowledgeable, concerned, empathetic, a good educator, and a good motivator, a diabetic patient, whether man or woman, will seek out such a doctor on a regular basis. (See Chapter 1, The Physical Man, for advice on how to choose a doctor for your diabetes care.)

June and Barbara: Earlier you pointed to stress as causing sudden dramatic rises in blood sugar. We realize that the stress that affects diabetics can be of two kinds: physical stress, such as a surgery, an infection, or being overweight, or emotional stress, such as a death in the family, a divorce, or the loss of a job. Could you explain why blood sugar is so seriously affected by stresses of both kinds?

Dr. Lodewick: Stress initiates a neuroendocrine response that sends messages to the central nervous system. The nervous system then acts on the endocrine system (glands) to release a variety of hormones—cortisol, adrenaline, glucagon, growth hormone, and others. These are known as *counterregulatory hormones*. They can raise blood sugar significantly. They cause an increased production of sugar (glucose) by the liver and a decreased uptake of sugar by the muscles.

I often see stress causing elevation in blood sugar in patients undergoing surgery or having some other major medical condition. In these circumstances, stress may even cause diabetes to develop transiently for the first time. Such people may temporarily need insulin. Once the medical or psychological stress is over, diabetes may disappear and blood sugar may return to normal. If the person has diabetes in the first place, the effect of stress is magnified greatly.

The subtle role of stress is perfectly exemplified by the story of a professional golfer I know.

THE STRESS OF THE GOLFER

Many people think of golf as a relaxing sport with plenty of walking for exercise and therefore ideal for stress relief. You'd think that it would be the perfect sport for the diabetic. And it probably would be, were it not for the competitive element in golf that causes stress rather than relieving it. One diabetic professional golfer, Ray Pelligrini, tests his blood sugar five to seven times a day, taking multiple doses of insulin to keep his diabetes control excellent. His blood sugars are frequently on par with his golf scores—high 60s to low 70s. And he has normal glycohemoglobin levels to prove the steady excellence of his control.

Ray says that when he goes out for a casual, noncompetitive 18 holes, he frequently finds his blood sugars lower because of the exercise and relaxation. However, when he goes for a competitive match (he hopes to make the PGA tour), the mental stress really affects him. Although he eats the same amount of food and gets the same amount of exercise, he finds his blood sugars go higher. He will even give himself an extra dose or two of insulin out on the golf course to keep his blood sugar controlled.

June and Barbara: You might tell Ray Pelligrini for us that we had the identical experience with golf, even though the thought of making the Women's PGA tour never entered our minds. Since competing just with Barbara causes June's blood sugar to go up, we solved the problem in a way that would probably appeal only to women: we stopped keeping score.

This brings us to the heart of the matter. Since you can't avoid most stress—it's a normal part of everyone's life—how do you change your reaction to it so that it won't send you out of control? When we sought answers to this question for June's sake, we found almost nothing written specifically for diabetics. So, after doing a great deal of homework, we wrote *The Diabetic's Total Health Book* in 1980, which addresses stress in a diabetic's life. We then revised it in 1988 when the destructiveness of stress in our society and environment had been recognized in medicine and new therapies were being offered. On a newsstand we recently saw a magazine featuring the headline, "Stress, the Major Illness of the 1990s." It looks like stress is here to stay.

Since stress is a double whammy for a diabetic—you have the usual stresses everyone has plus the stress of a chronic disease—it pays to get yourself into some methods of counteracting your counterregulatory hormones that send your blood sugar up. To reduce physical stress on your body, it is very important to have a good diet. And your diabetes exercise program works equally well as a stress-reducing program (provided it's not competitive professional golf). We can't praise exercise too highly in this respect. As you've related to us through your own experience, Dr. Lodewick, exercise releases endorphins in the brain, those hormones that do the opposite of the counterregulatory hormones and produce that familiar runner's high (see Chapter 4, The Sportsman). The endorphins are known as "the morphine within," which aptly describes what they do for a man under tension.

The exercises you can learn to perform with your mind are just as good for relieving stress as those you do with your body. Some of you may already be familiar with these techniques. For example, in one type of biofeedback you are hooked up to electronic instruments that check your temperature, pulse, muscle tension, and the speed of your brain waves. Using this information, you are taught to control these internal body processes through "cultivated relaxation."

Almost all of you have probably heard of meditation as a way of arriving at a tranquil state of mind. Other techniques you can learn through books or in classes are autogenics (self-hypnosis), progressive relaxation (tightening and then loosening all the muscles of your body), and visualization or guided imagery. These last two involve forming images in your mind to calm yourself. Even something as simple as the breathing exercises practiced in yoga can lift you out of a stressful situation and return you to a state of calm. Choose one of these peace-inducing activities, practice it until it works for you, and then take a few moments each day or whenever you feel the need and allow yourself the time to do it. It's as simple as that.

The above activities (or nonactivities) are what you might call mental minivacations. We find that real vacations work just as well. In spite of the old saying to the contrary, you can leave your troubles behind. We've met many businessmen who have learned that unless they get away from it all on a regular basis, they suffer burn-out, and instead of helping their businesses by overworking themselves, they harm them with their poor performance. Obviously, a diabetic man has even more to risk by locking himself into this kind of workaholic syndrome. So go away for a day or a weekend and see the difference in yourself and in your blood sugar levels.

From June's past experience with chronic headaches (non-diabetes-related), we suspect that physical pain can act as a stressor and can raise blood sugar. Have you seen this happen in your patients or yourself?

Dr. Lodewick: The question of pain is a tough one. Pain can directly or indirectly affect blood sugar control. Pain is an indication that some malady has affected part of the body or that some part of the body has been injured. The pain is caused by inflammation of the nerve fibers at the site of the injury. These inflamed nerves relay messages to the spinal cord and up to the brain. The neuroendocrine response—the same one that stress activates—then comes into play and sends out the counterregulatory hormones that raise blood sugar. The magnitude of the response occurs proportionally to the degree of the injury.

Pain can indirectly cause an elevation in blood sugar in several ways. It can cause limitation of physical activity so that you're not using or burning up as many calories, and those extra calories raise your blood sugar. Pain can also cause depression and stress because a man can't continue to do all the things he might otherwise be doing. It slows him down. And depression and mental stress stimulate the same neuroendocrine response that pain itself does, thus creating a vicious circle.

June and Barbara: Do you think one of the reasons men may have a different attitude toward their health in general and their diabetes in particular may be because male children are treated differently from female children? By this we mean socially treated, not medically treated. Are boys expected to tough it out? Be more independent? Are they given responsibility for their own care more than girls? Are girls more coddled by parents?

Dr. Lodewick: As I pointed out before, boys are ordinarily taught not to cry and not to be afraid, while girls are allowed to weep and are comforted when they express fears. But after a child is diagnosed diabetic, I think the parents should take the same approach whether the child is a boy or a girl.

As one of my patients puts it, "You can't buy it away, pray it away, wish it away. You have to learn to live with it." In fact, the way a child responds to diabetes may be asexual. A girl may rebel as much as a boy in the tough adolescent years. It's a matter of personality, not sex.

June and Barbara: We've seen plenty of evidence of that. By way of illustration, here's a letter we received from a 21-year-old woman who had just read our book, *The Diabetic Woman*, and wanted to tell us the story of her diabetic life. We've decided to include it here because we thought it might give The Psychosocial Man some insight into anger, denial, and rebellion.

I was diagnosed as having diabetes when I was 7 years old. That was 14 years ago, and lots has happened in those 14 years, most of it bad. I rebelled against anything having to do with diabetes from the day I was diagnosed. I was determined to be normal, no matter what happened. My mother was the enforcer who made me eat the gross food and test my urine daily. I was so terrible about sneaking sweets that my parents began to discipline me when I would sneak goodies. This made me rebel even more against most adult figures. The adults were always saying, "Jackie, should you be eating that?"

I hated all of my doctors and nurses. I really detested the dietitians. When I was 10 I began smoking and chewing tobacco. When my older brother caught me and told my parents, they were flabbergasted. They were at their wits' end. They talked to my doctor, a pediatric endocrinologist, about all of this. He was slightly concerned, but said, "This too shall pass."

I went to a diabetic camp when I was 8 and 9. My parents took me when I was 10, but I threw a fit and refused to stay! I really hated camp. It was too medically oriented. I just wanted desperately to be "normal," and I couldn't figure out how. Nothing I tried worked.

When I turned 13 I refused to go to a doctor anymore. I had decided I could control my own diabetes without people being on my case all the time. This actually worked out pretty well for me. I would eat whatever I felt like and then take the insulin needed to cover it. I still follow this plan, although I'm beginning to change.

My diabetes was virtually unnoticeable all through high school. Believe it or not, I only had real problems with ketoacidosis when I was 10. I only experienced one problem during my early teens and that was from food poisoning.

Anyway, on to where "I saw the light." I got a summer job after my senior year in high school before starting college. My problems began there. I began having severe hypoglycemic reactions at work. MAJOR EMBARRASSMENT!!

I decided I should see my specialist again. So after 5 years, I went back to the same pediatric endocrinologist. I was 17 at the time. He talked to me about testing and how important it was. I said yea, yea, and walked out of his office just as rebellious as when I had seen him the first time at 7.

I started college and met a best friend, a fellow diabetic. It was really cool because we had the same philosophy about diabetes: "Act like it doesn't exist!" I went low twice within a month. Both times I was unconscious and was hauled out of the dorm by paramedics. More MAJOR EMBARRASSMENT!!

My friends still tease me about missing homecoming my freshman year because I was in the emergency room. Even after these lows, I still kept plugging along like the big D wasn't a part of my life. My Resident Director and Resident Assistant wanted to talk to me about it, and I refused.

I knew what I was doing was wrong, but I was in a rut. I never kept my appointment with the doctor. My friends would bring me out of a reaction quite frequently, especially after a drinking party. I was either going to the bathroom constantly and drinking gallons of liquid, or I was passed out from being too low. I couldn't reach a happy medium.

This went on until this summer, when things began to change somewhat. In July a syringe needle broke off in my leg. No big deal, that's what I thought. I never had real problems in my leg until September. This was my senior year of college and I had to drop out. After numerous infections and six surgeries on my thigh, the needle is out. I am still fighting infection, and I still have one open wound in my leg.

I've been hospitalized six times since August. In August I had a severe reaction while driving my car. I passed out, ran a red light, and T-boned another car. I was trapped in my car for 45 minutes while they cut me out. Miraculously, I was not seriously injured and neither was the other guy.

I spent four days in the hospital then. This gave me a lot of time to think. This is when I started to realize how stupid I had been. I hadn't even turned 21 yet, and my life was a mess. I could have been killed, and worse, I could have killed another person. An innocent person could have been killed because I am selfish and stubborn. If I had been killed, I would have deserved it, but if I had killed someone and I lived, I couldn't have dealt with that. Older middle-aged people, friends of my parents, thought

I should have my license revoked! I wasn't too sure they were wrong!

Anyway, I made it through the wreck and returned to school, only to be back in the hospital a month later. This was when the diabetes nurses and educators started talking to me. I was still rebelling, even though I knew how ignorant and selfish I was being. One nurse dropped your book *The Diabetic Woman* on my table in my hospital room. She suggested that I read it. I laughed at her and said, "Sure, if I find time in my busy schedule!" Yes, I can be a smart ass, too.

I picked up the book a couple of times and read a few paragraphs. But I was so angry and unhappy that I couldn't read anything. I've had hospital stays of 4, 6, 7, 10, 9, and 10 days from August until December. A diabetic counselor's name was given to me about the third stay. I've been seeing her ever since, and I'm slowly being straightened out. I've seen my doctor and I have started testing with a meter four times a day. I feel guilty if I miss a time! I just bought three new books on diabetes, and yours was one of them. I really enjoyed reading it, and I will keep it as a reference when I need it. If you have any helpful hints or pamphlets on helping me get back on track, I would love to read anything you could send.

We did send Jackie what we could, and we have the feeling now that, having survived her hazardous adolescent years, she will protect herself from further diabetic mishaps and go on to make herself a rich and rewarding life.

Although we talk more about teenage sons in Chapter 9, Your Diabetic Son, we'd like to ask you a question here that applies to The Psychosocial Man. What do you think are the underlying reasons for this rebellion that all teenagers seem to go through, although not all of them to the degree of intensity and self-destruction that Jackie did?

Dr. Lodewick: Every teenager wants to cut the ties and become self-sufficient. Some more than others want to learn the ropes on their own through their own experience. Consequently, adolescent turmoil erupts in relationships with parents. Good parental advice often goes unheeded, much to the dismay of parents. The harder parents push to make their teenager do the right thing, the more the boy may rebel, even to the point of doing the very opposite or the wrong thing. This is done just to make the point that he's his own man, even if this means insulting his mother and father with cosmic fury.

Eventually the relationship may mature. The parents stop battling their child to steer him into the right and correct course, and they allow him to take the reins of his life himself. And the teenager may begin to realize that his parents are not his adversaries, and he may even (and this is almost beyond belief) permit them to give him advice or help him achieve his goals.

June and Barbara: When a teenage boy has diabetes, how does this complicate the rebellion?

Dr. Lodewick: This adds yet another serious dimension to the relationship. Parents become upset, worrying that their boy may ignore his health and doom himself to physical and mental impairments later in life. This happens unless the boy quickly learns how to care for his diabetes. Learning can be accomplished in several ways. He can read diabetes magazines and books, he can test his own blood sugar, he can consult with his doctor and talk with a nurse educator, and he can work with groups such as the American Diabetes Association, the Juvenile Diabetes Association, summer camps, and other youth support groups in his area.

To keep his parents off his back, he can prove to them that he is capable of getting good blood sugar results (between 80 and 160 mg/dl before a meal) and acceptable glycohemoglobins (7 to 10%). This relieves the strain immensely. A teenager can even set up a kind of contract with his parents to the effect that if he succeeds in getting good results, they will stop nagging about doing tests, eating right, and exercising.

Once good results are obtained, some teenagers will continue to take good care of themselves, as they will be happy that they've accomplished this difficult task. Others will learn more about their own human nature and realize that they are, in fact, dependent creatures and that it is a rare human being who can accomplish life's goals without the help of others. I found this out in my own youth. When I got diabetes, I knew I needed the help and support of many people. My friends and family, and today my wife and many of my patients, have made me see ever so clearly the need to care for myself. They have shown me that I could not do it without them. Teenagers who see themselves in this light may find it helpful to ask their parents to keep reminding them (NOT nagging them) to follow the straight and narrow path of good diabetes care.

June and Barbara: When a diabetic man is contemplating marriage, does the family of his bride-to-be sometimes create potential roadblocks because of his diabetes? One of the reasons we ask is that Rabbi Harvey J. Fields of the Wilshire Boulevard Temple in Los Angeles had such an experience. Writing in the *New York Times Magazine*, he told of falling deeply in love with a girl when they were both juniors in college. They corresponded constantly over the summer, making plans for their future together. Then in August she wrote that her parents wouldn't allow her to return to the university. Rabbi Fields described the situation: "Stunned, I called her. 'Why?' I asked. 'They don't want me marrying a diabetic,' she said tearfully. 'Dad says it's too risky, too many problems to take on.'"

Incidentally, he later married another woman and they now have three diabetes-free children.

Dr. Lodewick: I suppose some parents of the bride-to-be may be concerned that their future son-in-law is handicapped. This notion is based on their ignorance, of course. I remind you, there have been many great diabetic men, including Thomas Edison, Anwar Sadat, and Aaron Copland, who prove that this is a false assumption.

The parents may worry, too, that their grandchildren might have diabetes or be unhealthy. I'd advise them that this is not necessarily a concern, especially with good care. My own four children, ages 11 to 24, are good evidence: our 24-year-old daughter Tori is at the University of California at Santa Barbara; our 19-year-old son Matt is at the University of California at Berkeley studying premed; Pete, our 22-year-old son, is planning to make photography his career; and our 11-year-old daughter Sarah is terrific in all respects and a great tennis player aspiring to be the next Steffi Graf. No bad health and no diabetes among them!

Actually, I have not witnessed any of these in-law fears. Maybe that's my fault. When one of my patients is about to get married, I don't inquire about the concerns of his bride's family. If I know him as a good man, I am confident he will be a good husband regardless of his diabetes.

June and Barbara: Have you found many men who resisted getting married or having children because of their diabetes?

Dr. Lodewick: Most men don't look upon diabetes as a reason not to get married, particularly if they feel they are healthy, can manage diabetes, and know how to prevent the complications. These same men do not resist having children, as they know there is not a great chance of their children developing diabetes. But if this should happen, they know diabetes can be well controlled and probably even better controlled in the future.

On the other hand, as we've already alluded to, some men unnecessarily think of diabetes as a weakness. They think of themselves as being imperfect and unworthy and, therefore, not good enough for the woman they love. It is a mistake to think that nondiabetic men are superior to diabetic men. Or if diabetes has already caused physical problems, particularly if it has affected his heart or sexual system, a man may not want to burden his female partner with his medical problems and will resist marriage.

June and Barbara: Do fathers of young children have trouble revealing their diabetes to their children and relying on them for help on the occasions when they need it?

Dr. Lodewick: I've been impressed that most fathers do reveal their diabetes to their children, although they don't like to reveal it to the average lay person. This is understandable because of the way the average nondiabetic views diabetes. Since they have never come into contact with a diabetic, many people do not have the slightest idea of what it means to have diabetes, nor do they understand the intricacies of it or the individual differences between diabetics. The average nondiabetic, therefore, tends to categorize, misinterpret, condemn, or pity the diabetic out of ignorance.

Fathers don't have to be concerned that their children will react in the same way because their children love them and want to help. Fathers know they won't be condemned by their children. Their children won't think less of them as men when they see them accept the challenge of facing the problems of diabetes (unless, of course, their fathers totally disregard their diabetes).

My children knew of my diabetes from very early ages. My wife Maureen and I discussed diabetes frequently in front of our children. I am reminded of our oldest daughter Tori who, when she was four years old, was already familiar with the term "sugar in the urine." (That was in 1970 when diabetics evaluated their control by checking the amount of sugar in their urine.) Tori got sick to her stomach one night at 2 A.M. We heard her get up and go to the bathroom and vomit. We rushed to help her. Relieved of her nausea, she proudly told us that what she threw up "had no sugar in it."

Then years later, when I was a more experienced diabetologist, I was helped by my son Matt. He was 12 at the time and rode his bicycle with me while I jogged. One day after working all night at the hospital, I was dead tired but I still felt I needed to go jogging. I assumed I was tired from lack of sleep and a "hard day's night." I lugged myself along step after step and let Matt know of my fatigue. Matt suggested that I check my blood sugar. Sure enough, rather than lack of sleep, it was hypoglycemia that was draining my energy. Thereafter, I knew whenever I felt sleepy or tired to be sure to check my sugar to guard against hypoglycemia. I also learned that my athletic performances were better when I kept my blood sugar slightly over the ideal range of 120 to 150 mg/dl, especially before a long event.

I cannot leave out our youngest daughter Sarah. She's been helping me with my blood sugar testing since she was four or five years old. She also has plenty of questions to ask if I don't get my sugar in the reasonable range of 90 to 150 mg/dl, and she wonders why I don't do as well as she does, because when she tests hers it is always in the 70 to 110 mg/dl range.

Finally, I think that having my children know about my diabetes helps in other ways, too. Most important, I am motivated to show them a good example, which in turn motivates me to take good care of myself. In addition, though I am a doctor with diabetes, I am also human and I tend to make mistakes. They forgive me for this humanness. They also know that no one, not even themselves, can be perfect. However, they are always behind me, helping me toward keeping in the best of control, but allowing me to make occasional mistakes without being too critical.

Also, there is the potential for one of my children to develop diabetes. So far, my children are 24, 22, 19, and 11 years of age and show no indication of diabetes. Because they see that I am taking good care of myself and leading a full life, they know that if they did develop diabetes, they would not have to let it hold them back either.

June and Barbara: A phenomenon sometimes called "male menopause" may involve a man leaving his wife and taking up with a younger woman. Possibly the reason for this is a realization of your own mortality and the need to seize the day with someone younger who'll make you feel younger yourself. Does diabetes ever make men have that feeling of mortality at an earlier age or intensify it whenever it occurs, causing them to manifest similar symptoms? Along with that, are there any physical problems for male diabetics that may cause a mid-life crisis?

Dr. Lodewick: In menopause, women have a dropping off of estrogen and female hormone production. This can result in a number of symptoms including an acceleration of the aging process. In men, there is generally not a reduction in the male hormone testosterone until very late in life. This being the case, male sexual activity generally continues to run high from birth to grave, and it is only when there are problems in his marriage that a man may decide to take up with another woman. A man certainly wants to know that he is still desired, and a fulfilling sexual relationship best serves this purpose. The more mortal he feels, the more he likes this sexual relationship. Yes, diabetes definitely makes men feel more mortal at the age when diabetes first strikes, especially when they are over the period of denial.

However, men with diabetes generally have good male hormone levels and therefore have normal libido and enjoy good sexual relationships. In the many men I've seen with diabetes over the years, I've not been impressed that they develop unusual tendencies to run off with younger women, especially if they find strength in their marital union.

June and Barbara: Do you feel that a husband's diabetes sometimes puts a tremendous strain on a marriage?

Dr. Lodewick: I've certainly seen cases in which diabetes has severely put the marriage vows to the test, but in most of these cases the marriage was already in trouble for reasons other than the diabetes. The marital situation of one husband who was a patient of mine and his wife—we'll call them Mr. and Mrs. Jones—particularly comes to mind.

Mr. Jones was a dedicated man who worked hard and brought home a good paycheck. But he admitted to me that he was grateful he worked shift work, as did his wife, so he had a break from her ranting and raving. When he retired and they had more time together was when the real problems began. For one thing, he told me, she always had to be right. Of course, he realized the importance of self-testing of blood sugar and so he always performed the tests, but she demanded to scrutinize the results. When his blood sugar was high, she came down on him like a ton of bricks, pummeling him with "What are you cheating on?" and "What did you do wrong?" and other choice phrases of that nature.

Even though he was following a prescribed diet, her desire for his perfection led to relentless harassing attacks on him. To abate these attacks, you can predict what he did. He did just what an adolescent son, who is frustrated by an overbearing mother, would do to get her off his back. He falsified his blood sugar results. While in her company he was the most perfect of diabetic men. He was grateful when Mrs. Jones, who was still employed, went to work so that he could take a break from perfect diabetes control.

So here you have a marriage with deception and an acrimonious tug-of-war. On the surface it looks as if the diabetes caused their problems, but in reality it was just a handy weapon to use in their on-going battle. If it hadn't been diabetes, they would have found something else to wage war with.

June and Barbara: Have you seen any cases in which the marriage seemed in fair shape where the husband's diabetes— or at least the couple's reaction to his diabetes—caused serious problems?

Dr. Lodewick: Yes, I've seen quite a few relationships splinter because of the development of diabetes. This is more likely to occur if diabetes is diagnosed early in the relationship or marriage. One young man's wife described the situation in this way: "From the first day he was diagnosed, there has been a change in him. He's been sick all the time. He's not the same, he's so pessimistic. He lashes out. There's been a definite change in his personality. Yes, he works, but when he comes home, he just sits, drinks, and sleeps. He's not romantic anymore and his love life has gone out the window."

Needless to say, this woman dragged her husband in to see me, hoping that I might have some insights into what caused all these changes after he became diabetic. He seemed blithely indifferent to his wife's analysis of his condition. But he subsequently admitted in private conversation that his sexual desire and ability had left him six months before. This man had never accepted his diabetes. He rejected it, at least in the sense that he was not doing anything to keep it under control. His poor control, in turn, may have contributed to his being depressed, sapped of energy, and unresponsive to his wife. This relationship, in my analysis, was on the brink of disaster. It could be saved only if he made a major effort to stop ignoring his diabetes.

So, as we have seen, a marriage can be rocky if the wife has perfectionistic tendencies. Here the husband has no room for mistakes. Because there can be no perfection when you have diabetes, these relationships are filled with resentment and dissatisfaction. I've seen many of them dissolve. The wife's constant harping on her husband to do everything exactly by the book—diet, exercise, four to six blood sugar tests a day—makes him feel like a child and fills him with resentment. His reaction may be to totally ignore his diabetes. However, if he is caring for himself, educating himself, testing himself, and keeping himself appraised of the pros and cons of good and bad control, there should be no need for his wife to play any more than a supportive role and the relationship should flourish.

The opposite can also happen. The downfall in a relationship may stem from a perfectionistic tendency in the diabetic man. There is one man I've known for years who has always had an intense desire to keep his blood sugars "perfectly" normal (70 to 110 mg/dl). The only problem was that his schedule was erratic, and he didn't want to change it because he preferred a varied schedule. In addition, although he wanted and strived for perfect blood sugars, his hunger and desire to eat would always overcome his desire to keep perfect blood sugars, and as a result he would often overeat. This overeating would naturally cause his blood sugars to rise, and not wanting to have them high, he would give himself extra insulin. This, in turn, would cause moderate hypoglycemic reactions. During these low blood sugar periods, he was extremely hostile and cantankerous to all those around him. His fiancée became increasingly frightened and alarmed by this behavior. As a last resort, she urged him to seek my help one final time. She delivered the ultimatum that unless he followed my advice and avoided these constant insulin reactions, she was leaving him.

I outlined a program for him and forbade him to take extra insulin to get his blood sugars back down after overeating. But since he was a perfectionist in matters of blood sugar, he couldn't stand seeing them high and persisted in giving himself extra insulin. When hypoglycemia was the inevitable result, his fiancée packed up and left.

Finally, there's the story of the young man whose wife was in the throes of divorcing him because of his workaholic habits and the limited time he could spend with her and their two children. When he developed diabetes, this was further complicated by the psychological trauma he suffered. The wife described how diabetes changed him. He had always prided himself on how healthy he was, never missing a day's work and working seven days a week, putting in 12 hours a day. After he was diagnosed with diabetes, he was always complaining. He imagined he was having heart symptoms and that his low blood sugar was causing him to be weak and dizzy, although he could never document low blood sugar with a test. He was bothered by choking, which both he and his wife described as ''relentless.'' Emergency room and doctor's visits never found a physical cause. His wife urged him to consult me.

As did his previous doctors, I told him all these symptoms could well be psychological. I explained why he had them. He had been scared by the diagnosis of diabetes. In his mid-30s, he had felt before the diagnosis that he had many years to slow down and give his family more time and romance. Now he was doubtful. He fancied that diabetes would abbreviate his life and that the thrill of success at work and in marriage would pass him by. He felt guilty at not having spent more time with his wife and growing family. I reassured this man and his wife that he was healthy and could well live a long, active life. I told him that he should make a major attempt to curtail his workaholic schedule and that his wife would be satisfied with him even if he weren't Number 1. After this marital/diabetes conference, I sensed that there was a deeper understanding between them and that the relationship would change for the better.

POSTSCRIPT

Keeping Company with Diabetes

As we look back on this chapter, we can see that many of the questions and answers we dealt with often fell more into the social than the psychological area. Our unabridged *Random House Dictionary* gives several definitions of the word *social: pertaining to, devoted to, or characterized by friendly companionship or relations; seeking or enjoying the companionship of others; living or disposed to live in companionship with others.*

You can see that the term *social* covers a multitude of relationships with your spouse, partner, family, friends, associates, and even casual acquaintances. Relationships, involving as they do interactions with other human beings and their foibles and idiosyncrasies, are always complex and confusing.

What happens when you add your constant companion diabetes to the equation? It can make no difference at all—or it can make a huge complicating difference. It's like introducing a new person to an established member of your social network. Diabetes, just like a person, can be immediately accepted by your family and friends. Or it can be regarded with fear, suspicion, hostility, or surprisingly, even jealousy, because diabetes is taking so much of your time and attention—time and attention that was formerly devoted to them. They may feel that diabetes is an unwanted intruder, a spoiler of fun, something like an unpleasant and incompatible person whom you drag along everywhere you go.

Some people may pretend your diabetes isn't there in an effort to not let it encroach upon their lives or yours. Others may bend over backward, being overly solicitous of the unwelcome guest—but you can tell that in their heart of hearts they don't like diabetes at all and wish it would just go away and let them enjoy your company without its interference.

You'll have to face the fact that some members of your social network will never come to terms with the sometimes intrusive presence of diabetes, even as certain friends may never accept your choice of a wife or some childless individuals will never welcome your visits when you bring along your disruptive offspring. But most of your intimates, those who really love you, will, after a period of initial shock and confusion, settle down and accept your diabetes and come to regard it as just a part of you like your hair—or lack thereof.

The clue as to whether or not you gain this acceptance of your diabetes from others lies in your own attitude toward it. Do you understand it and accept it in a matter-of-fact way? Do you try to make it fit unobtrusively into your life—and theirs? And when it causes problems, do you keep your perspective and your sense of humor about it and work out those problems in a calm and rational way? Or do you resent its presence and constantly complain about how impossible it is, how you hate it, and how it's ruining your life? Your attitude, be it positive or negative, will very likely become theirs. Only you can make your diabetes socially acceptable.

The
TRENCHERMAN
. . . .
Real Men Do Weigh Their Food

A few years ago there was a humor book written by Bruce Feirstein called *Real Men Don't Eat Quiche: A Guidebook to All That Is Masculine.* As is often the case with humor, there was much truth in his delineation of stereotypically masculine products and activities. He particularly hit home on the food section. There are sexual implications in the foods you eat and the drinks you drink—and even the way you eat and drink them. This book pointed out which wimpy foods—besides quiche—that Real Men don't eat: pâté, poached salmon, tofu, yogurt, asparagus, broccoli, arugula, salad, light beer, crêpes, lemon mousse, and so on. On the other hand, Real Men eat the likes of bacon cheeseburgers, frozen peas, watermelon, French fries, pretzels, and apple pie. Their drinks run along the lines of beer, Jack Daniels, and Gatorade. Presumably, they wolf down and gulp down prodigiously gross quantities of these in the manner of Henry VIII or Diamond Jim Brady or William "The Refrigerator" Perry.

Thus it has been down through history. In his book, *The Physiology of Taste*, Jean Anthelme Brillat-Savarin noted that in medieval times it was believed that a man's appetite was in direct proportion to his importance. You could recognize a real heavy-hitter in those days when he was served "no less than the whole back of a five-year-old bull and his drink in a cup almost too enormous to lift."

Women have been known to contribute to masculine sexual food stereotypes. We've heard women announce with pride almost as if it were proof of her husband's sexual potency, "My Joe will eat anything as long as it's steak and potatoes."

Younger men—especially those seriously involved with sports—and more enlightened older men are managing to escape from this macho menu trap and eat healthily, selectively, intelligently, and moderately. Still, most men so detest having to bother thinking about eating the right foods at the right times that they frequently just give up and head for the nearest fast food chain for a quick fix or eat whatever's available at a restaurant without considering any of their special needs.

If it's any comfort, most diabetic women dislike all this preoccupation with food—keeping snacks on hand, weighing and measuring portions, and worrying about dining times—as much as diabetic men do. But women are more likely to do it, anyway, docile, compliant creatures that they are. (How's that for a sexual stereotype?)

For all diabetics, however, care and concern with good nutrition that results in improved diabetes control is a necessity—and can be a virtue. If you put into practice the knowledge you gain about healthy eating, you will not only do much toward keeping your blood sugar normal, but you will also feel, look, work, and play better. Your change to an improved diet may also educate and inspire your family members and friends to improve their way of eating. That way you'll have company in your new dining habits as well as the company of your longer lived family members and friends throughout your life.

By the way, real diabetic men *shouldn't* eat quiche. It's full of fat and cholesterol.

—June and Barbara

W H A T   Y O U ' L L   F I N D   H E R E

DIABETIC DIET (TYPE I AND TYPE II)

SKIPPING MEALS

FIBER

CALORIES

LIQUID PROTEIN DIETS

MAKING DIETARY CHANGES

CHROMIUM

VITAMINS

ALCOHOL AND DRIVING

June and Barbara: You would think that diet would be the easiest part of the diabetic treatment plan since we all have lots of experience eating. But we've found the opposite to be true: diet can be the most complex, confusing, and neglected aspect of diabetes control. Do you agree with this?

Dr. Lodewick: Yes, and a survey by the National Institutes of Health indicated the truth of it. They found that the majority of people with diabetes fail to control their diabetes by diet alone. This is a shame because most diabetes specialists would agree that in more than half the people with Type II diabetes, diet can be the deciding factor in whether insulin or oral agents are needed. Controlling excessive food intake lowers cholesterol and blood fats and may help prevent heart and vascular disease. Even people who must use insulin for control need to avoid overeating to prevent consistently high blood sugars, which may cause lethargy, weakness, fatigue, and even more serious symptoms.

June and Barbara: If diet can work all these wonders, then why do so many people fail?

Dr. Lodewick: In the same National Institutes of Health survey, it was cited that as many as 20% of people with diabetes have never gotten any diet information at all, another 20% didn't understand their diet, and another 40 to 60% didn't follow their diet, most likely for social reasons. From this, it's easy to see why the failure rate with diets is so high.

This has been the experience that I've seen over and over again with people who have come to me for advice. They had been given a *diet list* and told to follow it. The information on these lists is informative for some, but many do not understand it. Unless a man understands a diet or a meal plan and how it helps with the treatment of his diabetes, he may very well reject it.

To improve upon this failure rate, I believe it's crucial for men with diabetes to understand their dietary requirements and to integrate them successfully with some luscious foods into their way of life. Food, after all, is not just sustenance, it's also pleasurable and social. What social event (dating, weddings, funerals) or even business affair ever takes place without food serving as a medium between people? Yet these important social aspects of food are overlooked when a man is confronted for the first time with diabetes and a diet sheet on which only one thing is considered—diabetes control. But just as important is that the teenager can eat with his buddies, that those with religious or ethnic requirements can partake of special foods or can fast, and that an older person can enjoy a favorite meal with his friends.

By understanding some basic nutritional information, men can satisfy all their basic food needs without sacrificing either general health or the diabetes diet. Food can be proportioned and varied so that men maintain their ideal weight, strength, and vigor while controlling blood sugar and fats. Food can still pique the senses of smell, taste, and sight and be an integral part of life's daily events.

June and Barbara: One of the most controversial topics in the treatment of diabetes, and a question we are asked constantly, is "What is the best diabetic diet?" How do you handle this hot potato?

Dr. Lodewick: The medical literature is rife with pros and cons for many different diabetic diets, each proponent of one or the other plan championing different proportions of carbohydrate, fat, and protein and each dictating the type of carbohydrate, fat, and protein that should be eaten. Some recommend a low-carbohydrate, high-protein diet such as Dr. Richard K. Bernstein, author of *Diabetes: The Glucograf Method for Normalizing Blood Sugar,* and Dr. Atkins, author of *The Diet Revolution.* The good point about Dr. Bernstein's recommendation is that he does obtain excellent blood sugar control, but the diet entails very hard work with frequent blood sugar testing. Also, the large amount of fat in the diet (40%) may not be healthy from the standpoint of heart and vascular disease. The same criticism goes for the Atkins diet of very high fat and minimal carbohydrate. Not that all types of fat are bad for a person, as there is some indication that fish fat (omega-3 fatty acids) may not be as damaging as animal fat. (Eskimos consume a high-fat fish diet, yet have little arteriosclerosis or heart disease.) But the meat and egg diet of Dr. Atkins goes too far.

More and more, however, the medical literature is steamrolling toward the diet of Nathan Pritikin (the Pritikin Program); Dr. James Anderson, author of *Diabetes: A Practical New Guide to Healthy Living*; and yours truly, Peter A. Lodewick, author of *A Diabetic Doctor Looks at Diabetes, His and Yours.* We all favor a high–complex carbohydrate (50 to 60%), low-sugar, low-fat (10 to 20%), low-protein (10 to 20%) diet. Preferably, there should be less than 200 to 300 mg of cholesterol consumed each day. In 1984, results of the Oslo Heart Study and the Lipids Research Coronary Prevention Trials were reported as showing a marked reduction in heart disease resulting from dietary changes to lower cholesterol.

As a consequence, more and more physicians are recommending diets similar to the ones Pritikin, Anderson, and I have been
recommending for years.

There are certain situations, however, where a lesser
percentage of carbohydrate may be advisable. Excess carbohydrates, even if complex, will elevate blood sugar. Unless you
can prevent yourself from overeating spaghetti, lasagna, or
other foods loaded with "carbos," it may be better to limit the
amount of carbohydrate in your diet, particularly if you are a
Type II trying to do without insulin. In this case, only about
40% of your calories should come from carbohydrate, 40%
from fat, and 20% from protein. Dr. Lois Jovanovic-Peterson
recommends a similar diet distribution for some of her
pregnant women to avoid the blood sugar elevating effects of
excessive carbohydrate.

As you can see, to some extent the diet depends upon
your goals. To simplify, I prefer to talk separately about diets
for Type II diabetes and those for Type I diabetes, because diets
that will work to normalize blood sugar for Type II's are not
identical to those for Type I's.

June and Barbara: Since most men are Type II's, why don't
we consider their diet first.

Dr. Lodewick: Let's start out with an example of a man who
came to me with Type II diabetes and how I changed his diet
to control his blood sugars.

THE CASE OF THE BOTTOMLESS STOMACH

George definitely had the most gargantuan appetite I have ever
seen. By age 38 he had achieved a solid weight of 300 pounds.
His friends affectionately referred to him as "the garbage
disposal, the food processor, the bottomless stomach, the
empty leg," and a number of other insulting, yet accurate,

names. Unfortunately, this propensity to eat led to difficulty: it activated his genetic tendency toward diabetes and he ended up with 500 mg/dl blood sugars.

In analyzing a patient's condition, a dietary history is of great help. It's my routine to review these histories to see if I can determine whether a man is a big, average, or small eater. There are many overweight people who are *not* big eaters. Small eaters have a tougher time getting their blood sugar down by dieting because they already don't eat that much. With this information, I can make a clinical hunch as to whether someone can manage without the need for insulin. With George I could stop analyzing his dietary history at breakfast. Before noontime rolled around, he had already consumed 4000 calories! He told me it was his custom to have three breakfasts: one at home, another on the road, and one when he got to work. Here is George's morning menu:

HOME		ROAD		WORK	
Breakfast No. 1	**Cal**	**Breakfast No. 2**	**Cal**	**Breakfast No. 3**	**Cal**
10 pieces of toast	420	1 omelette	420	3 doughnuts	600
6 pats of butter	240	2 muffins	320	4 cups of coffee	
6 eggs	420	2 servings jelly	80	8 tsp. sugar	160
6 strips of bacon	270	2 pats of butter	80	4 oz. cream	180
1 qt. orange juice	400	2 cups coffee			
4 cups of coffee		4 tsp. sugar	80		
8 tsp. sugar	160	2 oz. cream	90		
4 oz. cream	180				
	2090		1070		940

This grand total of over 4000 calories was combined with several other meals during the day. It wasn't unusual for him to consume 10 pork chops or 10 hamburgers at one sitting. The analysis of such a voracious appetite had several helpful implications. There was no doubt in my mind that with a reasonable diet, George's blood sugar would get within the normal range and he would have no need for insulin. He was definitely a big eater—in contrast to many other overweight people who are victims of a sluggish metabolism and/or an inactive lifestyle and are small eaters. By the simple task of dropping his calories to a reasonable 1800 to 2000 per day, within three weeks his blood sugars returned to normal. A small eater couldn't cut back that much on calories because he wouldn't be eating that much to begin with.

If George stays on the path of dietary righteousness, I have every confidence that this ''cure'' of his diabetes will be permanent. I've seen many men who, if they continue to be careful with calories, keep their blood sugar in the normal range for years at a time.

However, I must warn you not to get too lax. Many Type II men have a tendency to start ignoring their diet once the scare of the onset of diabetes is over. They are feeling well and their blood sugars are back to normal. They add a piece of cake here and some ice cream there. Some even return to guzzling beer. But don't be fooled into thinking that just because your blood sugar is normal after overeating, this means overeating is not a problem. Before long, you will become fatter and fatter and again run the risk of having your diabetes go out of control. The second time around, your blood sugar may not improve as much as the first time simply by returning to your diet, and medication, including insulin, may be needed. Not only that, but even if blood sugars don't become elevated above the 140 mg/dl range, you must remember that overeating is not only bad for diabetes and the heart, but it can raise blood fats and accelerate the aging process, which no man likes to face. In some men overeating can do all this without even causing any symptoms or giving any clues.

Here are some maxims to remember:

Overeating is bad for diabetes.

Overeating causes heart disease.

Overeating accelerates the aging process.

Overeating may raise cholesterol and triglycerides.

Many men have never realized the detrimental effect over-eating can have and, because they may feel pretty well despite high blood sugars and blood fats, they continue to overeat. I generally recommend a number of books that highlight the need to restrict food to preserve health. One of Nathan Pritikin's books, Covert Bailey's books, or Dr. James Anderson's books are very helpful in this regard (see References).

June and Barbara: What's the special importance of diet for Type I men and how does taking insulin affect how they eat?

Dr. Lodewick: In learning about food, a diabetic man on insulin must realize that the constituents of his daily menu can cause quite a fluctuation in blood sugar control, depending on the type of insulin he's on and how often he takes it. Although it is important to know how food affects blood sugar and cholesterol in Type II diabetes, in general you don't see the marked fluctuation in blood sugar that you do in insulin-dependent diabetes. For example, in Type II diabetes, overeating 100 to 1000 calories may cause blood sugar to be 300 mg/dl at 7 A.M., 330 mg/dl at 11 A.M. and 330 mg/dl at 5 P.M. In some Type I diabetics, however, blood sugar might go from 100 mg/dl to 700 mg/dl and back to 100 mg/dl in the very same day, depending on the type of insulin he uses and the frequency of injection.

Conversely, if a Type II man skips food, this may not cause much of a drop in blood sugar, while skipping as little as a single starch/bread exchange (80 calories) for a Type I diabetic could mean the difference between a good blood sugar of 110 mg/dl and a poor blood sugar of 40 mg/dl associated with an intense insulin reaction. Thus, it's important for these "brittle" (unstable) men, particularly if they are trying to get as good control as possible, to know the calorie content and especially the carbohydrate content of the meals they are eating. (Carbohydrate is more significant than calories in raising blood sugar in Type I diabetics.) You should distribute these carbohydrates and calories as evenly as possible throughout the meals of the day to match your insulin dosages and avoid the peaks and valleys of high and low blood sugar.

Also, it is important for Type I's (as well as Type II's) to know the "glycemic index" of foods (see Appendix D). This index is a classification of how high and how fast certain foods raise your blood sugar. It shows that different foods that have basically the same carbohydrate and calorie content can cause a markedly different rise in blood sugar. The index lets you choose foods that tend to stabilize blood sugar rather than escalate it suddenly. Unfortunately, it only covers 62 foods, but even so, it is helpful in deciding what to eat.

June and Barbara: You mentioned the danger of skipping meals. Could you amplify this point? We find there's a lot of confusion about whether you can or can't skip meals or snacks when your doctor or dietitian has assigned them to you on a daily eating plan. In fact, we've been amazed while teaching people blood sugar testing at the SugarFree Center that even though the meter has just shown them that they have a blood sugar of, say, 290 mg/dl, many of them will look at their watches and say, "Oh, my gosh, it's time for my snack," and want to get up immediately and go buy something in our food store or pull something out of their briefcase to munch on. When we try to explain that eating food while their blood sugar is 290 mg/dl will simply run that high figure up even higher, they don't seem to comprehend. They defend themselves by saying, "But this is when I was told to eat my morning snack." It's almost as if all logic has left their brain, and they have been preprogrammed into senseless behavior. Often it's impossible for us to keep them from committing the folly of sending their blood sugar even more out of control.

On the other hand, some men who want to or need to skip a meal because of an important business meeting or an emergency find themselves in a dilemma. How can this be handled—or *can* it be handled at all?

Dr. Lodewick: The answer depends on the kind of diabetes the man has and whether he takes medication. Considering Type II diabetics first, if the man is not on any medication and calorie restriction is strongly recommended, then skipping a meal is fine, especially if home blood sugar tests are over 180 to 200 mg/dl. Make sure, however, that blood sugar is not over 300 mg/dl or associated with very poor control, which may in fact reflect insulin deficiency, as blood sugars with poor control may go higher even without eating.

For Type II men on oral medicines, the danger of hypoglycemia is always there, especially if they keep their blood sugar where it should ideally be, that is, in the normal range of 80 to 120 mg/dl. Sometimes men taking oral medicines regularly overeat and have chronically high blood sugars, so occasionally skipping a meal will not provoke hypoglycemia. The main danger for these men is not low blood sugar, but the toll that chronically high blood sugars may be exacting on their vascular systems.

The story is somewhat trickier for men with insulin-dependent diabetes. It's important for them to avoid hypoglycemic or insulin reactions. It's true that I have a number of patients who skip breakfast after taking their insulin in the morning. The reason most of them can get away with this is that their blood sugar upon arising is high: 200 to 300 mg/dl or more. They know this because they test their own blood sugar. It takes several hours for their blood sugar to drop back into more reasonable (not hypoglycemic) ranges, especially if they are taking intermediate-acting insulin (Lente or NPH) or long-acting insulin (Ultralente). These men are safe from insulin reaction because they know their blood sugars are high and can risk not eating without provoking hypoglycemia.

In contrast, the better controlled men on insulin with blood sugars in the more normal range can't skip meals because they know that skipping may provoke low blood sugar reactions. The exception to this is the person on an insulin pump who takes multiple injections and closely monitors his blood sugar. He can cleverly learn to be more flexible about when to

eat and yet maintain good control. This would also apply to
men who use the basal–bolus method of insulin injection
described in Chapter 1.

On the other hand, for the man prone to insulin reactions
or with brittle diabetes, especially if he doesn't monitor his
own blood sugar carefully, it is very chancy to skip meals. I've
too often seen the result: a trip to the emergency room with
some serious consequences.

June and Barbara: We also want to point out that both
Type I's and Type II's should be aware of the role of fiber in
diabetes control and health. We are fiber fanatics ourselves—
bran, cereals, beans, whole fruits, and vegetables—all the
good-for-you foods that fill you up, not out. Fiber cannot even
be digested by the human body. One kind of fiber (water
insoluble) merely adds bulk and makes you feel full and
satisfied but does not put on weight. The other kind (water soluble) is slowly absorbed and helps prevent the rise of blood
sugar. Equally important, soluble oat bran and pectin fiber
actually lower blood cholesterol and triglycerides. These three
advantages are especially important for you diabetic men. And
we haven't even mentioned the fact that fiber is a preventive
influence on such health problems as cancer of the colon,
colitis, and constipation.

So try to include more high fiber foods in your diet. In the
American Diabetes Association's *Exchange Lists for Meal
Planning*, high fiber foods are indicated by a little wheat stalk
so that you can easily identify them. Try to eat 25 to 40 grams
a day if you can. If you can't get them in your food, you might
do as Barbara does (her father had cancer of the colon): take
a fiber supplement each day (Fiber Xcel or Fiber Supreme).

Along with fiber, another key issue for every diabetic
man—Type I or Type II—is how many calories to eat. How do
you find this out?

Dr. Lodewick: A dietitian or your doctor should assign you the proper number of calories, as it varies for each individual. There are big, medium, and small eaters, as we mentioned earlier. The purpose of calories is to maintain an ideal weight and provide the daily energy requirements. Parents of diabetic children are particularly concerned that their young ones are getting enough calories. The parents of one young man were concerned because he was so thin and was hungry despite eating 4400 calories a day. As it turned out, he was thin because his diabetes was out of control, and after reducing his calories by 1000 and adjusting his insulin, he gained weight.

An example of how few calories are needed even for great athletes is exemplified by Mr. Universe, Tim Belknap. He developed diabetes at age 14 and by 17 was still a scrawny 110-pound weakling. Then as described in Joe Weider's *Muscle and Fitness*, in June 1986, he got into nutrition. He now follows a healthy complex carbohydrate diet with only 1800 to 3200 calories per day, depending on the amount of exercise he anticipates. That's a relatively small number of calories for such a large, muscular athlete.

June and Barbara: So how do you gain the necessary knowledge to calculate your daily calorie intake? Lots of men are mystified by calorie calculations.

Dr. Lodewick: Again, you have to seek out the help of a dietitian or nutritionist. He or she will familiarize you with the *Exchange Lists for Meal Planning* published by the American Diabetes Association and the American Dietetic Association. You'll be taught how to read food labels and how to incorporate some of the canned, boxed, and frozen foods into your daily menu if convenience is important to you. You'll learn that calories come from only three basic sources: protein, carbohydrate, and fat. There are four calories in one gram of protein, four calories in one gram of carbohydrate, and nine calories in one gram of fat. Knowing this, you can estimate from the food labeling how many calories there are in each serving. Let's take milk, for example. An eight-ounce glass of whole milk has

12 grams carbohydrate (12 × 4)	= 48 calories
10 grams protein (10 × 4)	= 40 calories
8 grams fat (8 × 9)	= 72 calories
	= 160 calories

Whereas, an eight-ounce glass of skim milk has

12 grams carbohydrate (12 × 4)	= 48 calories
10 grams protein (10 × 4)	= 40 calories
	= 88 calories

You can see that eight ounces of whole milk have about twice as many calories as skim milk just because of the added fat content. For a man who drinks a quart of milk a day, this can mean a difference of 300 calories, depending on whether it is whole or skim. For the man who wants more variety of fat, these 300 calories could instead be in peanuts, butter, or mayonnaise, or the fat could be eliminated and the calories used to provide carbohydrate and protein. Remember, though, if you do this, the extra calories of carbohydrate and protein may have a higher glycemic index and cause a higher blood sugar than fat. To help determine if there is a higher glycemic index, self-testing of blood sugar is of paramount importance. Then, with your doctor's help, you can determine whether a slight increase in insulin dose is needed for the extra carbohydrate and protein. And even though fat doesn't raise the blood sugar as much as carbohydrate, it's still important to test blood sugars to make sure insulin requirements are not *diminished* with decreased calories.

June and Barbara: It always makes big news when celebrities such as Oprah Winfrey lose a lot of weight on one of those liquid protein diets. Then there are even bigger headlines when they put it back on again—often gaining back more than they originally started with. What's your opinion of the efficacy of these diets? Do you recommend this kind of diet for overweight diabetics?

Dr. Lodewick: Bariatricians (those who understand and treat obesity) have recognized for many years that there are many overweight people whose caloric intake is minimal. In other words, there are a lot of small eaters who are obese. It has been the misconception of many in the medical profession that overweight people eat much more than thin people. Physicians even use such derogatory terms as the "hollow leg syndrome," which ridicule their overweight patients. However, studies of patients in university settings now indicate that there are many overweight people who do not overeat. In one very interesting study reported in the *New England Journal of Medicine* (February 28, 1988), it was shown that some infants of overweight parents also become overweight at three months of age and that this could be explained by the fact that their bodies expended much less energy.

For the adult who eats sparingly and for those who are metabolically out of control, very low calorie diets are finally being increasingly recognized as sound therapy—at least until the medical condition is under control. For overweight diabetic patients, blood sugars may return to normal even without insulin. Their blood fat content may also be reduced. However, there are some caveats to be aware of.

When the very low calorie liquid protein diets such as the Cambridge Diet first became available, the protein amino acid composition was inadequate and possibly lacking in minerals such as potassium. This could promote a loss of muscle mass, even of the heart muscle, causing dangerous disturbances in the heart rhythm and, in some cases, death.

Today the composition of these diets is better, with adequate protein derived from milk or eggs. All the daily requirements of minerals and nutrients are also supplied if taken properly. Most medical authorities feel, however, that these diets should only be dispensed under a doctor's advice and supervision. Frequent medical check-ups and laboratory testing are considered essential. Needless to say, to follow a very low calorie diet properly, there is considerable expense involving doctors, nurses, dietitians, and sometimes even psychologists to help with behavior modification.

As you point out, although very low calorie diets are successful with initial weight loss, long-term results have been very disappointing. That's one of the reasons why a man might need to have recourse to behavioral modification techniques. These should include a long-term maintenance program in which he is educated or re-educated in weight management strategies for controlling extra calories that contribute to being overweight.

We should also mention here what is now called "yo-yo dieting" or "the yo-yo syndrome." Many overweight people find that, after initial success in losing their desired weight, they rapidly gain it back. Then, the next time they try to lose the weight, they find it harder to succeed even on the same restricted diet and will regain the weight even more rapidly when they slip off their diet, which they invariably do.

Research studies of obese people and laboratory animals indicate there is a change in the metabolism that causes increased difficulty in losing weight each time a person goes back for another try. To compound and aggravate things even further, when they do regain weight it is frequently distributed more to the upper body than to the lower body. Upper body weight gain has been associated with an increased risk of heart disease, particularly in men.

My advice, therefore, is to avoid this yo-yo syndrome so you don't have to face the increased risk and difficulty in losing weight. Make a determined commitment to change your eating habits gradually but permanently in association with regular exercise. Become motivated to be healthy. Follow the example of

Richard Simmons, one television personality who has managed to keep his weight off. Of course, his motivation may be a little different than yours—the success of his fame and fortune with his books, tapes, and TV shows depends on his keeping his weight off!

June and Barbara: Changing your diet, especially if it means restricting yourself, is not an easy thing to do, even for a reason as valid and serious as diabetes control. Do you have any tricks of the trade to help men make these changes?

Dr. Lodewick: It's rare for anyone to be able to fight the food battle alone. The problem for the food eater is not like the smoker's or the drinker's problem. As long as the smoker doesn't take the first smoke, he won't smoke; as long as the alcohol drinker doesn't take the first drink, he won't drink. For the food eater, however, it's a totally different story. He has to eat to survive, so as soon as the first food comes along, it poses the possibility of overeating, whether it be a simple peanut butter sandwich or chocolate mousse de quoi. For example, if a person's diet says that he should eat only three-fourths of a peanut butter sandwich and you place a whole one in front of him, you can bet he will eat the whole sandwich. For some, this small extra amount may make the difference between a normal 120 mg/dl blood sugar and a 160 mg/dl.

In my experience there are several techniques that will help · a man stick to a reasonable diet. First, as we mentioned, you have to learn the calorie contents of different foods. After that, one of the most helpful techniques is to keep a food diary. Many men find they are eating many more calories than they ever thought, often unconsciously. Listen to how one man found out he was overeating.

JOHN WEARS A SURGICAL SCRUB MASK

John loved cooking for friends. It was not until he had the nifty idea of wearing a surgical scrub mask over his mouth that he found evidence of many blocked attempts at food sampling while he cooked. There were food stains all over the mask, much, I imagine, like the unfaithful lover being found out by lipstick on his collar.

A food diary is even better. It helps determine if there are certain triggering factors causing overeating: stress, anger, boredom, depression, time of day, and so on. Then with this realization, work on methods to avoid the overeating that comes from such factors as stress and time of day. You'll soon be able to analyze your bad habits. Do you eat any time there's food in front of you? Do you eat so fast you consume a gigantic meal in five minutes—and then begin to eye the plate hungrily as if you might want to eat even that? The way the eating diary has helped many men with diabetes has led to what are now considered the Ten Commandments of Eating by many eating behavioralists, as well as myself.

The Ten Commandments of Eating

1. Thou shalt not eat just because you are upset, bored, or depressed.
2. Thou shalt not consume sweets, for this desire stems from craving, not hunger.
3. Thou shalt take time out for eating.
4. Thou shalt eat slowly to taste the food and give the brain the chance to say "enough's enough."
5. Thou shalt eat slowly to allow for some communication among the food participants, especially important for the talkers of the group.
6. Thou shalt not clean the plate.
7. Thou shalt confine eating to the dining area.
8. Thou shalt keep tempting foods that you are trying to avoid out of sight or preferably out of the house.

9. Thou shalt not take the first bite of a forbidden but desired delicacy or you won't stop.

10. Thou shalt keep plenty of healthy food available and in sight.

(Actually, there are more than ten commandments for eating. I highly recommend the book *Habits Not Diets* by James M. Ferguson, M.D., for more details.)

June and Barbara: As women we're afraid that we have the typical prejudice in that we feel men have a harder time learning about food because the kitchen and cooking have always been female territory and women grow up knowing more about cooking recipes and meal planning. (We realize, however, that most chefs of famous restaurants are men.) Do you have examples of men who have taken charge of their diets and worked out perfect control of weight and blood sugar?

Dr. Lodewick: Well, I have one example, but I wouldn't recommend his technique. As a Type I diabetic, he fully realized the importance of diet. So he learned what worked for him and he began to eat the exact same thing every day, and I mean the *exact* same breakfast, lunch, and dinner. He did this for over 30 years! Every day he brought a banana, a thermos of milk, and a meatball sandwich with him on the road, as he was a traveling salesman. He cooked the meatballs the night before to ensure that he got the same amount of meat in the sandwiches each day. Although he certainly did a good job controlling his blood sugar and was free of any major complications, I think he could have done just as well by spicing things up a bit with a little variety.

You men can learn food values and how to plan appropriate meals just as well as women. Food knowledge is power. In fact, the more you know about food, the less restrictive you have to be with your daily schedule. By knowing the approximate number of calories in the food you like, you can adapt your eating schedule to one that suits you. You *don't* have to eat supper at 5 P.M. or else. You *can* eat at 4 P.M. or 8 P.M. or any other time, as long as you know how to avoid hypoglycemia by having an appropriate snack or making adjustments in your insulin dosage. You can also decide which diet you prefer, be it vegetarian, high-carbohydrate, low-fat, or whatever. When you dine at a restaurant, you can learn to choose from the menu with greater confidence. There is even a new book out called *The Restaurant Companion* by Hope S. Warshaw, which covers virtually every kind of restaurant menu and gives calorie estimates and exchanges for all of them.

June and Barbara: Unlike many physicians, you rarely seem to accuse your patients of cheating on their diets. To us this is a refreshing attitude, and we wonder why you came to drop the accusatory manner that other professionals use in dealing with people who are not too successful with their diabetes management.

Dr. Lodewick: Let me give you just one example of a man who came to me because his eminent endocrinologist had accused him of being a cheat. This physician had assigned Phil a diet of 1800 to 2000 calories a day and Phil did his best to follow it. When his blood sugars did not come under control, the physician prescribed oral agents and finally insulin. Despite a large dosage of insulin, Phil's blood sugars did not come down. He felt miserable and became thin and weak. When his endocrinologist labeled him a "cheat," unhappy and annoyed, Phil came to me.

In evaluating his condition, I was impressed that, although he was probably eating a little more than the 1800 to 2000 calories he had been prescribed, he should not have had such poor control nor should he have been losing weight on 100 units or more of insulin. To ensure that my analysis was right, I placed him in the hospital on 1800 calories a day. I found that his blood sugars remained very high, despite my further raising his insulin dose to over 120 units. I then realized that it was not his diet that was at fault, but that he could be resistant to the relatively impure beef–pork insulin he was taking. Upon switching Phil to purified pork insulin, I was able to drop him to only 45 units and his blood sugars dramatically improved. He felt better and regained the 20 pounds he had lost on a relatively restricted 1800-calorie diet. He was not a "cheat."

June and Barbara: Phil was a lucky man indeed to have found you to diagnose his problem so astutely. Many men go from doctor to doctor without finding a solution to their own difficulties with diabetes. Feeling just as desperate and defeated as Phil, they latch onto whatever medical information or misinformation they find in popular magazines and try to do a little self-medication. One of these "miracle" solutions to high blood sugar that keeps popping up is the alleged benefits of the mineral chromium and what it does for the control of diabetes. Is there any validity to these recurring claims about chromium?

Dr. Lodewick: Chromium plays a critical role in the proper utilization of sugar in the blood. Chromium deficiency results in resistance to the effect of insulin, just what a diabetic does not need. A chromium deficiency can thus make the blood sugar go higher, particularly in Type II diabetics. In fact, in some patients, restoring sufficient chromium will control Type II diabetes, especially if the diabetes is mild and of recent onset. It's estimated that between 50 and 200 micrograms (a microgram is one-millionth of a gram) is needed in the diet to prevent chromium deficiency. In general, there are only about 25 micrograms for every 1000 calories a person eats, so that for many non-insulin-dependent men on restricted diets of less than 1500 calories, chromium deficiency may exist. For these men, 10 to 15 grams (a generous tablespoon or two) of brewer's yeast can be used as a supplement to prevent chromium deficiency. Good food sources of chromium include whole grains, peanuts and peanut butter, apples, prunes, plums, and American cheese.

Type I men, especially if on low-calorie diets, may also suffer chromium deficiency. This may result in resistance to the effect of insulin so that higher doses are needed to control blood sugar. By restoring their chromium levels to normal, insulin-dependent men may need less insulin.

Finally, chromium can have beneficial effects on blood fats, both overall cholesterol and "good" cholesterol (HDL). Since these levels are frequently disturbed in diabetes, men should ensure that they get an adequate chromium supply (but not an oversupply) through diet or supplementation.

June and Barbara: Here's another controversial one for you. Should diabetic men take extra vitamins?

Dr. Lodewick: When the word "vitamin" is used, ears perk up. What are they and how crucial are they to giving men the four V's—virility, vitality, vim, and vigor? This is a heated topic of debate from eminent people on both sides of the issue. Physicians who have the greatest experience and who are the most thoroughly trained in the management of disease are scathingly criticized for their "ignorance" of nutrition and vitamins.

Gabe Mirkin, M.D., who wrote the *Sportsmedicine Book*, could hardly be considered ignorant in this regard. An expert in the field of nutrition and exercise, he stands on one side, feeling that an adequate diet should provide sufficient vitamins without the need for supplements. Nathan Pritikin, famous for his program for cardiovascular fitness, stands on the same side, indicating no need for supplementation despite his low-fat, low-protein diet, which is relatively low in vitamins. It's hard to argue with Pritikin, because when he died at age 69, an autopsy showed virtually no evidence of hardening of the arteries or arteriosclerosis. Richard K. Bernstein, M.D., author of *Diabetes: The Glucograf Method for Normalizing Blood Sugar*, and Dorothea F. Sims, author of *Diabetes, Reach for Health and Freedom*, both of whom have had diabetes over 40 years, also do not express the need for large vitamin supplements. At the largest center in the world for the treatment of diabetes, the Joslin Diabetes Center in Boston, doctors are also reluctant to recommend big vitamin doses.

On the other side of the issue is the winner of two Nobel prizes, Dr. Linus Pauling. His recommendation of using massive doses of vitamin C sent the nutritional world into a tizzy. Despite no scientific support to document his argument that 2000 milligrams or more of vitamin C should be used each day to prevent colds and possibly cancer, he has had enormous influence. (He must be doing something right, as he is now 90 years old.) Millions of dollars per year are now spent on vitamin C.

Joining Dr. Pauling in the need for vitamins are many chiropractors and nutritionists who diagnose vitamin deficiency (I'm not sure how) and then recommend various supplements. It's not uncommon for me to see men who come from these nutritionists' offices consuming up to $220 worth of vitamins a month. Some of these men become very ill, possibly because of the toxic effects of the vitamins. Many of them feel much better when they stop taking them.

In my experience as a physician, having seen over 3000 patients with diabetes, I am not convinced that vitamins have made any difference in the ability of patients to avoid the vascular complications of diabetes. Some live 50 years with diabetes despite the fact that they don't take vitamins, may even smoke, and have poor blood sugar control. Others soon have vascular complications despite vitamins, a good diet, and attempts at good control. The answer may reside more in the susceptibility that each individual has toward complications. That is the answer we are looking for—why some people are more susceptible than others to the complications of diabetes.

While we search for this answer, it may be that vitamins and minerals should be added to the diet, especially if it is a low-calorie diet or a high-fat or high-fiber diet. (Fiber interferes with vitamin absorption.) While many diets are sufficient in supplying the FDA's Recommended Daily Allowance (RDA) to prevent a specific vitamin deficiency, some experts speculate that much higher allowances are needed for an anti-aging effect and possibly other protective effects. To be more specific, although the RDA for vitamin A is 1000 units needed to prevent vision loss, some say that 10,000 units may be necessary to protect against vascular disease and possibly cancer. Charles Hennekins of Harvard Medical School, for instance, thinks that beta-carotene, a substance found in many fruits and vegetables which is converted to vitamin A by the body, has an anticancer effect. He is studying this possible effect in 22,000 doctors. Half the doctors are taking 50 milligrams of beta-carotene daily and the other half are not. Being one of the participants in this study, I am anxious to see the results.

Inositol (a B vitamin) may prevent neuropathy in uncontrolled diabetes when taken in much larger doses than the RDA. Many also suggest that higher doses of vitamins A, C, E, and some of the B's may be helpful for their anti-aging effect. Possibly the one who has put the vitamin controversy in best perspective is Sheldon Hendler, M.D., Ph.D. In his book *The Complete Guide to Anti-Aging Nutrients*, he suggests that the common people have to be pioneers in the use of vitamins for their possible but not proven anti-aging and health effects. Until that controversy is finally resolved, he recommends the daily consumption of the following vitamins:

Vitamin	Daily Amount
Vitamin A	20,000 units
Vitamin C	500 mg
Folic acid	400 μg*
Vitamin B_1	10 mg
Vitamin D	400 I.U.
Vitamin B_2	10 mg
Vitamin E	200 I.U.
Niacinimide	100 mg
Calcium	1000 mg

Vitamin	Daily Amount
Pantothenic acid	50 mg
Chromium	100 μg*
Vitamin B$_6$	10 mg
Copper	2 mg
Vitamin B$_{12}$	6 μg*
Selenium	200 μg*
Biotin	100 μg*
Iron	18 mg
Zinc	15 mg

(Reprinted with permission from *Prevention Magazine*, August 1985.)
*The unit μg is a microgram, one-millionth of a gram.

In the meantime, may each man have the four V's he needs—with or without vitamins!

June and Barbara: Let's move from vitamins to the vineyard. Classic trenchermen—the hearty eaters of days gone by—were often described in legend and song as being "jolly topers" or hearty drinkers, as well. But in the modern era the problems of alcoholism and driving under the influence are such that we no longer modify a drunk with happy-sounding adjectives. Although drinking is on the wane, it nevertheless remains a significant part of our culture. On a daily basis, many of us have to cope with situations in which alcohol is, if not a temptation, at least a social necessity. Could you outline for us some of the problems alcohol can cause for a diabetic man—in addition to the problems it can cause for a non-diabetic man?

Dr. Lodewick: It's true that a good percentage of men consider alcohol vital to their very social existence. Few are the social gatherings that do not include alcohol on the menu. In small amounts social drinking probably doesn't cause significant damage, but as the amount of alcohol consumed on a daily basis begins to creep up to much over two ounces, the trouble begins—especially for a diabetic.

Alcohol is a toxic substance that has many deleterious effects on your body and mind. These effects can include muscle aches, sleeplessness, anxiety, depression, diminished sex drive, increased cholesterol and triglycerides, liver damage, greater susceptibility to cataracts, osteoporosis (even in men), and gastrointestinal disorders. Heavy drinking does some of its most serious damage to your nervous system, where it causes neuritis and neuropathy (diseases of the nerves, which result in pain from inflamed nerves). Since nerve damage also occurs with out-of-control diabetes, the combination of alcohol and diabetes can greatly aggravate the neuritis–neuropathy tendency. At a recent annual meeting of the American Diabetes Association, they emphasized that diabetics consuming two to four ounces of alcohol per day have a much higher incidence of neuropathy than those who don't drink. So if you are a regular drinker, have your doctor check to make sure that neuropathy isn't present. In its early stages, neuropathy causes no symptoms. It can be there without your knowing it. You should have your doctor do this neuropathy check even if you are only a recently diagnosed diabetic. Research studies have shown that neuropathy can develop within one year of diagnosis. Even if tests reveal that no neuropathy is present, if you continue to drink—even just socially—you should have the doctor keep checking for neuropathy on a regular basis.

I have many surgical colleagues who don't drink any alcohol at all because they don't want their nerves damaged or their hands to be shaky when they're performing delicate and precise surgery. And I don't like my tennis shots affected, so I keep my alcohol intake to a minimum, which keeps my tennis opponents frustrated.

The acute effects of alcohol can be hazardous to your health if you drink much more than two or three ounces. In the early days of diabetes therapy, it was recommended that alcohol be substituted for food containing carbohydrates since alcohol doesn't take insulin to metabolize. But alcohol isn't a carbohydrate and doesn't perform like one in the body. It doesn't raise the blood sugar as a carbohydrate does. On top of that, alcohol inhibits the liver's capacity to make sugar from other nutrients in the bloodstream. Therefore, if alcohol is substituted for carbohydrates, it can have a double effect on lowering blood sugars. And since alcohol dulls your wits, if hypoglycemia does occur, your judgment is impaired and your ability to recognize and treat hypoglycemia may fail. This is especially true because the symptoms of hypoglycemia and the symptoms of the varying stages of inebriation may be indistinguishable from one another.

June and Barbara: It sounds from this as if the "don't drink and drive" admonition goes double for a diabetic.

Dr. Lodewick: It certainly does! With alcohol you are adding a third driving handicap to a person who already has to avoid hypoglycemia and may have impaired vision or reflexes as a result of his diabetes. Alcohol acts as a sedative to the brain. At first there is agitation, but then there is a rapid loss of self-consciousness, judgment, and self-control. The ability to think and recall diminishes. Associated with all this is an increased sense of skill and confidence out of context with reality. ("I can easily pass this car before the truck gets here.") The three D's of drinking, diabetes, and driving are a combination that can lead to a fourth D—death.

June and Barbara: A diabetic man can solve this drinking and driving problem by volunteering to be the designated driver when he goes out with friends. That way they'll consider him a great guy for taking on this burden and they certainly won't press him to join them in drinks as they might otherwise. Some restaurants in Los Angeles and other cities are encouraging the idea of a designated driver by rewarding him. In some cases, it's free nonalcoholic drinks or, alas for a diabetic, a free dessert.

But others go so far as to give the designated driver a whole free dinner. This makes it even more worthwhile to make the "sacrifice" of abstaining from alcohol.

As is often the case in talking about diabetes, we've thus far concentrated on the insulin takers. Does alcohol cause any special problems for people on diabetes pills?

Dr. Lodewick: Yes, particularly when you take Diabenese. When you combine that with alcohol, an Antabuse-like reaction can take place. Antabuse is a drug that was created for treating alcoholics. What it does is block one of the pathways of the metabolism of alcohol, turning it into an aldehyde (dehydrogenated alcohol), which sets off a violent physiological response including abdominal cramps, nausea, vomiting, diarrhea, and prostration. For people prone to this kind of reaction with alcohol and oral hypoglycemics—you have no way of knowing if you're one of these people in advance—you should beware of drinking alcohol with your pills.

June and Barbara: For the overweight diabetic there is also the problem of the heavy dose of calories you get from alcohol. Fortunately, there are some new alcohol-free wines—Ariél is the most widely distributed of these—that not only allow you to feel and look festive hoisting your glass, but have half the calories of regular wine. There are also a growing number of alcohol-free beers, but these often have as many calories and carbohydrates as the standard stuff.

Incidentally, calories and carbohydrates are important to watch for in anything you drink. Generally, Type I's should go for the low-carbohydrate products since carbohydrates raise your blood sugar, and the Type II's should look for products low in calories since calories put on weight. There are two handy pocket guides called *Snack Checkers* by Litestyler that will help with this (available for $10.95 + $2.00 shipping from Litestyler Systems, P.O. Box 9983, San Diego, CA 90340). *Snack Checker 1* lists, along with a number of popular snack foods, all the food values (including carbohydrates and calories) and exchanges for domestic, imported, and light beers. Using this, a Type I wanting to order a light beer would probably go for a Miller Lite since it has the fewest carbohydrates—2.8 grams (compared to Michelob Light's 12.4 grams). On the other hand, if you are a Type II who's concerned about weight, the choice would probably be an Olympia Gold Light, which weighs in at 72 calories, making it much lighter than Herman Joseph's Light's 130 calories or Michelob Light's 134 calories. *Snack Checker 2* performs the same service for wines and liquors as well as soft drinks, mixers, and juice drinks, plus a variety of snack foods.

At this point we should probably discuss another major hazard associated with alcohol—the classic hangover. Is a hangover particularly damaging for a diabetic?

Dr. Lodewick: If the acute effects of alcohol intoxication and/or associated hypoglycemia don't cause a catastrophe for your diabetes control, then a wicked hangover looms over you like a great buzzard. The dizziness, vertigo, nausea, vomiting, and headache of a horrible hangover can be so severe that they will wreak havoc with your diabetes. The stress of such a tumultuous condition can raise the blood sugar, but the inability to eat food can lower your blood sugar and confuse you to the extent that it's impossible to figure out the amount of insulin you should take and so you may not take enough. If this situation causes you to enter into the life-threatening state of ketoacidosis, you may wind up in the hospital for intravenous fluids.

June and Barbara: No amount of the so-called fun of a wild drinking party would be worth this trade-off! Considering what alcohol can do to a diabetic, you'll hate yourself for much longer than just in the morning if you overindulge, and you'll be a lot jollier if you are not a toper.

P O S T S C R I P T

Lunch Counter Intelligence

Time Magazine recently reported that CIA analysts believe that Mikhail Gorbachev is, as they call it, "a mild diabetic." According to their findings, he's had the disease since his 40s and he controls it with oral hypoglycemic tablets rather than insulin. They also theorize that his strong dislike of vodka and his campaign to keep consumption of it down in the Soviet Union is at least partly a result of his own need to avoid liquor—and watch his diet—because of his diabetes.

It's a comfort to know that if you should be elected President, you won't have any trouble following your diabetic diet at summit conferences with the Soviets—at least as long as Gorbachev is in power.

The
SPORTSMAN
· · · ·

Playing Your Way to Better Health

Exercise—and by this we mean fun and games—is great for what ails you. In fact, it is one of the basics of diabetes control. When the American Diabetes Association was founded, one of the interpretations of the pyramid logo they adopted was that it stood for the three components of diabetes control: diet, medication (insulin or oral hypoglycemics), and exercise. Unfortunately, back in those days, exercise was almost always neglected and that's why the pyramid of control so frequently collapsed.

Actually, neglected is too weak a word. More likely, exercise was condemned as dangerous for diabetics. For instance, back in 1928 when future tennis champion Bill Talbert was in the fifth grade, he was diagnosed diabetic. He tried to put an optimistic face on things by telling the nurse in the hospital how his new diet would improve his baseball playing by helping him run the bases twice as fast.

The nurse's stern reply was, "Now we can't have any of that, young man. Plenty of rest, that's what we're going to need from now on." This admonition was undoubtedly left over from the days before insulin was discovered and one treatment for diabetes was a near-starvation carbohydrate-free diet. The patient on this diet had to be kept inactive because if he exercised without carbohydrates, he'd have to use his own limited store of fat and protein for energy. We now know that if an out-of-control diabetic (over 250 mg/dl blood sugar) exercises, his blood sugar goes even higher.

Even as late as 1977 when we wrote *The Diabetic's Sports & Exercise Book*, there was little endorsement from the medical community for exercise as therapy and little information on how to go about becoming an athletic diabetic. We had to go directly to physically active diabetics themselves to find out how it was done. Fortunately, we were able to find 158 diabetic sportspeople, including several very successful ones, who loudly sang the praises of what exercise had done for their diabetes control. They even told us that diabetes, with its healthy regimen and necessity for self-discipline, had improved their sports prowess! When we asked in our lengthy questionnaire how these people had discovered the secret of successfully combining diabetes and exercise, they almost universally replied, "I learned by experience," "I learned on my own," or "I learned by trial and error."

Fortunately, the last few years have brought about a recognition of the value of exercise for diabetics. Now most diabetes education programs have an exercise therapist on staff to give direction to diabetics of all ages and conditions to get them into a regular exercise program. The arrival on the scene of blood sugar testing has probably played a major part in the acceptance of active sports for diabetics. Being able to know what your blood sugar is before starting the fourth quarter or plunging down the black double-diamond ski run or dropping off the side of a boat in your scuba gear has taken much of the fear and risk out of sports for many diabetics.

Exercise is one form of diabetes therapy that men usually take to better than women. Although this is changing, sports still remain much more a part of boys' and men's lives than they do girls' and women's lives. Take that natural inclination toward sports and run with it!

We discovered in our questionnaires from diabetic sportspeople something it took science a decade longer to recognize. Exercise is a wonder drug for diabetics. It accomplishes for you whatever particular needs you have. If you're a lean Type I diabetic who needs to put on some weight (or, more likely, muscle), exercise will put it on for you. This is because it works like invisible insulin to help you make use of the glucose that is converted from your food. If you're an overweight (generally Type II) diabetic, exercise will burn calories and help you lose those extra pounds. And whether you are Type I or Type II, it will help you keep your blood sugar normal.

When you come right down to it, if you have to have a disease, it's better to have one like diabetes because it gives you a good reason to go out and do what you'd like to be doing anyway. So play ball—or whatever your favorite sport may be!

—*June and Barbara*

WHAT YOU'LL FIND HERE

OUTSTANDING DIABETIC ATHLETES

MOTIVATION

ADJUSTING INSULIN AND FOOD (TYPE I'S)

BENEFITS OF EXERCISE FOR TYPE II'S

THE DAY-AFTER SYNDROME

PRECAUTIONS

STEROIDS

BODY BUILDING

OUT-OF-CONTROL DIABETES AND EXERCISE

FOOT CARE

EXERCISE AND BLOOD SUGAR CONTROL

June and Barbara: We know you are an enthusiastic and successful tennis player and runner. Have you been an active sportsman all your life, both before and after diabetes?

Dr. Lodewick: Yes. I've always loved sports and competition. This goes back to my heredity and the environment in which I grew up. I was born in Brooklyn, just a stone's throw away from Ebbets Field, the home of the old Brooklyn Dodgers. The time was the 1950s, the height of the Dodgers and the New York Yankees rivalry. My father was a former professional pitcher who at age 40 could still throw a dropball as well as Sandy Koufax.

My mother was also an excellent athlete. On top of that, I grew up with four other very athletic brothers in the alleyways of Brooklyn, where we would take on all challenges in the neighborhood whether it be fisticuffs, stickball, or any of the other numerous sports we engaged in. With this background, I was confident that I could face all of life's challenges—both sports and otherwise—and I have! Diabetes hasn't stopped me.

June and Barbara: Your diabetes never caused you any problems in sports?

Dr. Lodewick: Only very minor, short-lived, and easily corrected ones. For example, in a recent tennis match, diabetes *almost* got me into trouble. I started out in top form, building up a 6–0, 3–0 lead against one of my arch rivals. Suddenly, I was overcome by weakness. My legs began to wobble, my tennis strokes fell short, my concentration plummeted, and the score quickly took a turn for the worse. I dropped behind in the second set 3–4.

Fortunately, my wife Maureen was nearby watching this sudden turn of events. Recognizing that my sugar must be low, she offered me a Coke. I gulped it down, and the sugar quickly seeped into my bloodstream and re-energized me. My tennis opponent, who was temporarily beaming at the thought of a likely comeback, became despondent as my serves smashed in, my speed returned, my volleys became crisp and accurate, and my concentration again became keen. The game was soon over for my flabbergasted opponent.

June and Barbara: Not to discount your own superb amateur performance in sports, could you tell us if there are any professional or champion sportsmen who, in spite of diabetes (or maybe because of it), have made their mark as outstanding athletes?

Dr. Lodewick: There are so many examples of outstanding performances among diabetic men that I can only mention a few here. If we go back into the past, when good diabetes care was not even available, we find such men as Bill Talbert, U.S. National Tennis Champion; Jackie Robinson, first black to break into major league baseball; and Ron Santo, third baseman for the Chicago Cubs. More recently, we can name Catfish Hunter, great Oakland and New York Yankees pitcher; Bill Gullickson, former Montreal Expos pitcher; Bill Carlson, triathlon competitor; Pete Powers, M.D., marathon runner; and Jonathon Hayes, Kansas City Chiefs tight end.

As you can see from this list, these are top-notch athletes. The incredible performance of Pete Powers, who, with insulin-dependent diabetes, ran the marathon in 2 hours and 42 minutes is inspiring. He apparently consumed a concentrated sugar paste in a squeeze bottle every five miles. According to exercise experts, concentrated sugar prevents the stomach from emptying by possibly cutting down water absorption. Although you might expect this to have slowed him down, it didn't. In his case he needed it to get sugar to his muscles, and he no doubt succeeded in achieving this. The number of potential problems he overcame indicates what an outstanding athlete he is despite his diabetes. In fact, performances like his and many others that I've seen in my practice strengthen my suspicion that those who get diabetes when they're young are frequently better athletes than their nondiabetic counterparts. Getting diabetes is definitely not a reason to stop sports or exercise.

June and Barbara: In our *Diabetic's Sports & Exercise Book*, we discussed how many sportspeople agree with your sentiment that diabetics frequently become better athletes than their nondiabetic counterparts. Diabetes instills a sense of responsibility and self-discipline that carries over into sports training. The good health habits a well-controlled diabetic develops, along with a greater knowledge of food and nutrition, are further advantages for his physical conditioning.

Now that we know you're a physician who passionately practices what he preaches, maybe you could continue your sermon with a discussion of the additional benefits of exercise in case some of the men out there aren't True Believers yet.

Dr. Lodewick: The potential benefits of exercise are many. The idea that, ''Exercise is as good for the body as reading is for the mind'' has been well accepted by people who love both sports and intellectual endeavors. People with diabetes are no exception to this. In fact, exercise may even have a more beneficial effect on people with diabetes because statistically they suffer an increased risk of cardiovascular disease.

Some of the possible benefits of exercise include:

1. It increases sensitivity of body cells to insulin.

2. It helps with weight loss (if extra calories are not eaten).

3. It increases general physical fitness.

4. It decreases total cholesterol and raises the ''good'' (HDL) cholesterol.

5. It lowers blood pressures, usually by 10 to 20 mmHg.

6. It promotes the so-called runner's high, even if the exercise is something other than running.

For all of these reasons and if it's done under good medical supervision to help avoid some of the possible risks, exercise is highly laudable for diabetics. In studying over 17,000 Harvard alumni, Dr. Ralph Paffenbarger found that as calories burned during exercise rose from about 500 to 2000 calories per week, there was a steady drop in the risk of death. To burn 2000 calories per week, you'd need to run, jog, or walk an average of 15 to 25 miles.

June and Barbara: Maybe a good athlete such as yourself doesn't need motivation to exercise, but many men do. Do you have any suggestions on how they can motivate themselves?

Dr. Lodewick: Everybody needs motivation—even the super-stars. Knowing exercise is good and doing it are two different things. Despite all my knowledge of how it would benefit me, I still had a hard time getting myself to start jogging. That's where I needed the motivation. Several things urged me on. I was inspired by the magnificent writings of Dr. George A. Sheehan, reputed cardiologist, which stirred my competitive spirit. I was impressed that if Dr. Sheehan, who is no youngster, was running marathons and outdoing many a youth, I could certainly do as well. I was not even half his age. Dr. Sheehan is now in his early 70s, having taken up running in his 40s. Dr. Sheehan has a regular syndicated newspaper and magazine column. He writes the column ''Running Wild'' for the magazine *The Physician and Sportsmedicine*. He is the author of several great books on running and exercise (see References at back of book).

I've also been inspired by Dr. Kenneth Cooper, whose studies and writings show the protective value of exercise, and by Nathan Pritikin, who strongly recommends exercise in addition to his specialized complex carbohydrate diet.

However, in addition to these, I have had the good fortune to make the acquaintance of Dr. Zelcho Zic when we trained together in our diabetes fellowship at the Joslin Diabetes Center in Boston. He is the one to whom I owe so much for helping me develop the exercise habit. Zelcho and I used to play tennis a bit, but when winter in Boston came along, tennis was out of the question. Since he was an avid runner, he urged me to get off my duff and jog with him at the Brookline gym. That was a dreadful thought because I considered running painful and boring. But wanting to give him company in his drudgery, I acquiesced.

Then to make matters worse, he announced that we were going to run 44 times around the gym's tennis court (a circumference of 1/11 mile). He cajoled me more. He said that he was doing these 4 miles around the gym to "preserve my pancreas" because, as we both knew, exercise decreases the body's insulin requirements so the pancreas doesn't have to work as hard. Even with the admirable goal of pancreas preservation, I wondered how he managed to keep up this grueling running. Then I spotted his secret. He had a log book in which he recorded his mileage goals.

Date: January	4	5	6	7	8	9	10	11
Miles Run:	4	4	4	4	4	0	4	0

That made sense. He logged daily goals (4 miles), weekly goals (20 miles), and yearly goals (1000 miles).

I copied his secret. I set goals for myself. It appealed to my competitive spirit. If I set a goal, I knew I would accomplish it. However, I started out slowly. I didn't think I could start with 2 miles at a time, so I started with ½ mile, or 5 miles per week. It was hard at first, and I had my doubts. It was still drudgery as I built up to 1½ to 2 miles per day. I kept asking myself if this was really worth it. But my competitive nature prevailed. Finally, as I got over 2½ miles per day, I reached that renowned "runner's high." Then running became a pleasure. I'm now logging in 700 to 800 miles per year. The first ½ to 2 miles are no longer drudgery. In fact, now as soon as I step out the door, I'm in a state of tranquility and relaxation. Problems that would otherwise plague my mind are now answered easily as I proceed along the roadway step by step until I reach my goal.

Not only has running helped me in these ways, but as an added benefit, it has helped my performance on the tennis court by giving me more endurance. My game has gotten so good, for instance, that Dr. Zic, to whom I owe so much for getting me on the running road, will not even dare to challenge me to a tennis match.

In just the same way, I think that many of you diabetic men will succeed if you recognize the competitive spirit that lies within you. Everyone is competitive in the sense that he wants to succeed or be loved and praised, as psychiatrist William Glasser, author of *Positive Addiction*, would put it. Set goals, perhaps starting off with limited ones—½ mile walks instead of runs—and progress slowly. That way it won't be painful, and there will be plenty to gain as you feel stronger and more fit rather than weak and tired.

That's the story of how I found the motivation to run. But we're all different. You may find different motivations. For example, some of the reasons that motivate my patients to exercise include

To look handsome

To develop a good-looking body and legs

To improve sexual relationships

To improve general health

To lose weight

To meet companions

To relieve stress

To achieve a runner's high

To enjoy work more and be more productive, and

TO KEEP DIABETES IN BETTER CONTROL

To help keep you going in your exercise program try these ideas:

1. Set short-term goals of one week at a time. If you set goals, your basic masculine competitive urge should help you keep them.

2. Let your family and friends know what your goals are. They will help you see if you've fulfilled your pledge.

3. Don't set your goals too high. Start with limited goals and work up. In my case, for instance, I started with ½-mile runs and gradually built up to my present 4 to 6 miles, not thinking at the start that I could ever do that. However, I don't plan to run any more than this, as I believe it would be an unrealistic amount of time to set aside in my life just for exercise. Probably no more than this is needed for cardiovascular fitness.

4. Any exercise program you set up should be convenient to your home or work. That's why walking and jogging are so good for achieving your goals.

5. Give yourself a reward for achieving your goals. The best reward may be the knowledge that you are doing good things for yourself medically and physically, too. It also helps to praise yourself a lot when you achieve your goals.

June and Barbara: From our background in writing the *Diabetic's Sports & Exercise Book* and from June's own experience in adjusting her insulin and food during sports activities such as biking and skiing, we know that for Type I's at least, the trick is to judge how to alter food and/or insulin so that you can perform well and avoid low blood sugar. June has even done the opposite: miscalculated and ended up with high blood sugar. Can you give men some good advice for handling this?

Dr. Lodewick: There are so many factors involved that no man can always do this perfectly, as I've illustrated from my own mishaps. Before talking about the physiology of this, I must remind you that stress can play a major role in sports, too, as was shown by the story of the golfer in Chapter 2. It helps to know the exact effect of exercise on the body. Exercise causes the muscles and other tissues to need more calories, especially sugar, in order to do their work. Exercise also causes more insulin sensitivity, so that less insulin is needed to do its function of getting sugar into tissue and especially muscle. It's been well demonstrated in nondiabetics that the blood insulin level drops with exercise. There's a very sound reason for this. Less insulin means that low blood sugar will not occur to deprive the brain of its thinking capacity and the muscles of their maximum potential use. With low insulin levels, not as much sugar goes into some cells and the liver makes more sugar for immediate use instead of storing it.

That is what happens in nondiabetics, but in insulin-dependent diabetics the blood sugar level is not as perfectly adjusted by the body. The blood insulin level may not drop down because the insulin level is not determined by secretion from the pancreas but by the amount and type of insulin injected (Regular, NPH, Lente, or Ultralente) and the rate at which it is absorbed. The absorption rate depends on the type of exercise and the site of injection—abdomen, buttocks, arm, or leg. When the body is at rest, insulin is absorbed the fastest in the abdomen and next fastest in the arms and legs. But exercising the area where the insulin has been injected speeds up the insulin's action. And finally, with heavy exercise the injected insulin has more of a lowering effect on the blood sugar because exercise increases the effect of insulin—at least, in well-controlled diabetes.

So all of these factors—plus the variable factors of the vigorousness of the exercise, the toughness of the opponent, the duration of the exercise, and the temperature (on a hot day, the body has to work harder to cool itself off, which burns more blood sugar)—have to be integrated to make proper adjustments of food or insulin to allow for optimal performance.

Some recent studies indicate that when diabetes is out of control (blood sugars well over 200 mg/dl for a period of time), exercise will not *lower* but instead will *raise* your blood sugar and your athletic performance will be lackluster. It's my experience that this phenomenon occurs mainly in men who have an insulin deficiency and who therefore run *chronically* high blood sugars and may even be spilling ketones in their urine. Ketones in the urine generally indicate an insulin deficiency. Diabetics whose blood sugar goes inexplicably higher after exercise may not be taking enough insulin or their bodies may lack it.

Many men with diabetes will have a temporary high blood sugar (as high as 300 mg/dl), especially after meals, but they feel well and have no ketones in their urine (which is a sign of the lack of insulin). Their pre-meal blood sugars will run in the 80 to 160 mg/dl range. In general, these men should have reasonably good glycohemoglobin levels of less than 10%. So even if they have blood sugars of 160 to 240 mg/dl prior to the start of exercise, they will do well in their sport. Most of the very good athletes I've spoken to prefer to begin exercise with their blood sugars in the range of 120 to 240 mg/dl. As I mentioned previously, I make it a point myself to have my blood sugar above 120 mg/dl before I start a race or anticipate a long tennis match with a difficult opponent.

June and Barbara: Yes, you're absolutely right that the only way to begin exercise is to test your blood sugar and know that it's at a normal or above normal level. This gives a great sense of assurance. Then you can concentrate on what you're doing and not have to worry about getting that old familiar weak feeling and having to stop and eat, just when you don't want to. So now we come to the specifics of preadjustment of insulin and/or food. What are your guidelines?

Dr. Lodewick: For very heavy exercise of more than one hour's duration, most athletes prefer to eat less so that they don't exercise on a full stomach. For Type I men this means lowering the insulin dose so that insulin levels don't peak at the height of exercise. For nondiabetics, researchers have shown that insulin is needed but only in very small amounts during exercise. For insulin-dependent diabetics in good control, the dose of insulin that is peaking at the height of exercise may have to be reduced 20 to 70%. In diabetes camps for children where activity and varying strenuous games occur all day long, it is not uncommon to see the insulin dose of the campers reduced by as much as half despite no change in diet.

In my own case, instead of taking my usual pre-breakfast nine units of Regular on a day when I have an early morning tennis match, I may take only four to six units. This is why I like to take insulin four times per day—because it allows me to make an adjustment in insulin if an unanticipated tennis match or sports event comes up. I may not only lower the dose before the event, but even afterward, in addition to eating slightly more after a match as a guard against hypoglycemia. The following table gives a summary guide:

RECOMMENDATIONS FOR UNUSUALLY HEAVY EXERCISE	
Control	Keep blood sugar well controlled, with glyco-hemoglobin less than 10%.
Insulin	Drop usual dose that peaks at height of exercise by 20 to 70%.
Food	Same or slightly less, plus eat 10 to 25 grams of simple sugar every 15 to 30 minutes during exercise and extra food afterward.*
Blood sugar tests	Four to seven times per day, including before, during, and after exercise to help determine what level gives you the best performance.

*It was reported in the June 1990 issue of *Sports Medicine* that the Ross Laboratory product *Exceed Fluid Replacement and Energy Drink* (available in many supermarkets) does not raise blood sugar as much as simple sugars. It contains a complex glucose polymer that prevents rapid rises in blood sugar and may help to prevent low blood sugar after exercise. To see if it works, I plan to try this with my next anticipated marathon tennis match.

Before going ahead with any of these suggestions, discuss them with your doctor. Finally, I would like to add a special word of caution to Type II men who take oral hypoglycemics. The pills can cause hypoglycemia during exercise, and so you need to test your blood sugar whenever you feel your performance is lagging and eat a snack if necessary. You should also watch for low blood sugar after the exercise.

June and Barbara: We're glad you specifically mentioned the Type II's, since so far we've concentrated on the Type I sportsmen. What other suggestions do you have for non-insulin-takers?

Dr. Lodewick: Well, much of what I said about Type I also goes for Type II. Significant exercise lowers both the blood sugar levels and the resistance to insulin. As you remember, most Type II's have plenty of insulin, but it doesn't work right. Their insulin resistance occurs at the receptor sites on the cells (the muscle, fat, or blood cells). For insulin to be effective, it must attach itself at the receptor sites. If the receptor sites are defective or if there are not enough of them, then the body resists the effect of insulin. Regular and vigorous exercise cuts down on the resistance at the receptor sites to allow the body's insulin to work so that not as much is needed. Research studies on Type II diabetics show that after exercise, insulin levels are lower. Despite this lower insulin level, their blood sugars are better. And this is good, especially if my clinical suspicion is right—that the less insulin you need to get good blood sugars, the healthier it is for you.

The other major benefit of heavier exercise for Type II diabetics is acceleration of weight loss. A five-mile run may burn up to 500 calories during the run, but it may accelerate your metabolism for as long as 24 hours afterward so that even more calories are burned after you stop exercising. This is why exercise is particularly good for Type II overweight men. And since insulin is a fat-building hormone, the lowered insulin levels from exercise may help with weight loss in an additional way.

June and Barbara: Besides adjustments in insulin and food, what other measures may be needed for endurance exercise, especially in the heat?

Dr. Lodewick: WATER! Without water your body simply cannot function. Water accounts for 92% of body weight.

Although an average person can survive for weeks without food, death can occur within a few days without water. Your body loses an average of one or two quarts of water per day through your kidneys, lungs (exhaled as water vapor), bowels, and skin (through sweat). With heat and exercise, your body markedly accelerates its water loss by sweating up to as much as a quart or more of water per hour in an attempt to cool itself. If you don't sweat, your temperature goes up as heat is generated from your exercising muscles. For instance, marathon runners frequently have body temperatures of 104°F and higher. The body's temperature can even reach 106°F. This high temperature can cause the body systems to break down, and heat stroke and death can occur.

It's not easy to drink enough water to prevent dehydration during heavy physical exercise. With sweating and heat, your body can lose as much as two to four quarts of water, which equals four to eight pounds of body weight or as much as 5% of your total body weight.

Cramping may be the first sign that you are becoming dehydrated. If you don't replace water at this point, *heat exhaustion* occurs, manifested by dryness, nausea, and goose pimples with cold, clammy skin. If you don't stop and rest and drink some water, *heat stroke* may occur. At this stage, emergency hospital care is needed. To prevent this pernicious progression, DRINK WATER! One study reported that when one group was required to drink eight ounces of water every 15 minutes, they felt stronger and performed better than two other groups who drank nothing or drank only when they felt thirsty. Don't let thirst be the signal to drink. *Drink before you are thirsty.* In fact, keeping up with water replacement may be all that's needed for a non-insulin-dependent diabetic athlete on no medicine. The insulin-dependent diabetic may also need sugar or Exceed.

June and Barbara: We've heard some people recommend taking salt tablets when exercising in hot weather. Do you think it's a good idea to take those with your water?

Dr. Lodewick: No! They are dangerous during exercise because they cause the blood salt level to go even higher and may prevent absorption of water. Just plain old water is the key, at least for the man not taking insulin. The insulin-dependent man may need sugar, too, as mentioned in the previous question. (Test your blood sugar!) Drink one or two pints before exercise and keep drinking as much as you can tolerate throughout the exercise period.

Remember, though, if the temperature and humidity are both above 80, you may not be able to keep up with the demands, and it may be wiser to sacrifice a victory on the tennis court—as intolerable as that may be—than to risk heat exhaustion.

June and Barbara: You mentioned that exercise burns calories even after you stop. Could you elaborate on this phenomenon? Every diabetic sportsman needs to be aware of this for more reasons than one.

Dr. Lodewick: Exercise continues to lower your blood sugar and enables more calories to be burned off for up to 24 hours afterward. This phenomenon is known as the "day-after syndrome," and it's important to be on the alert for it to prevent hypoglycemia. You may need extra food because your body continues to burn up sugar. To find out if you do, test your blood sugar, or at least do a sensitive urine test every two to four hours after cessation of unusually heavy exercise. If your blood sugars are below 90 mg/dl, or your urine tests are negative, you may require an extra 10 to 25 grams of complex carbohydrates every four hours.

Another way to prevent the day-after syndrome is to incorporate the same amount of exercise into your schedule every day. Intermittent exercise is what leads to insulin reactions if you're not careful, as illustrated in Stuart's story.

BIOCHEMIST PLAYS BASKETBALL

Stuart is a biochemist so he was naturally interested in keeping his own biochemistry—that is, his own blood sugar—as close to normal as possible. At age 27, having had diabetes for four years, he was doing a good job of keeping his urine sugar tests negative (this was before the days of self-testing of blood sugar). However, one holiday season he got into the family spirit by playing three hours of basketball with his brothers. This was far more than he customarily exercised. He had no trouble during the game (his team won), but the next day he passed out at work from low blood sugar. After being given some glucose, he rapidly recovered to his usual fine self, but he was quite embarrassed.

June and Barbara: What are other possible dangers with an exercise program?

Dr. Lodewick: Excessively heavy exercise can definitely provoke a heart attack—especially in someone not in good physical condition. But people in apparently good physical condition can still have severe heart conditions and possibly not know it. Even marathon runners (such as Jim Fixx, who died during a run) and other athletes (such as Jack Kelly, Grace Kelly's father and an Olympic rowing champion) may not be exempt from heart problems. It is important to make sure you are in good medical condition before engaging in strenuous exercise. Hardening of the arteries is no doubt present to some degree in anyone over the age of 40 who has been on a typical American diet or even on what was (until 1980) the traditional American Diabetes Association diet consisting of over 40% fat. What has to be emphasized is that a person can feel well and yet have significant heart disease. If such a person, *especially* if he is out of condition, suddenly takes on heavy exercise, it may cause a heart attack. This is exemplified by one of my patients who, playing only a weekly game of men's doubles tennis, decided instead on a singles match when two of the foursome didn't show up. He had a heart attack on the tennis court. Fortunately, I arrived on the scene soon after and he survived, but he subsequently needed considerable care.

Other intermittent exercise that may create problems is lawn mowing and snow shoveling. If you're going to partake in such heavy work, make sure you're in shape first. Remember, people with diabetes frequently have silent heart disease; some even have heart attacks without knowing it, as the symptoms (chest pain, arm pain, or angina) are frequently not present. It's crucial to have a good physical evaluation and possibly even a stress electrocardiogram along with an exercise prescription before embarking on a course of heavy physical exercise. (See more discussion of this subject in Chapter 1, The Physical Man.)

You have to exercise consistently enough to condition your heart and cardiovascular system until you are in a state of physical fitness. This is referred to as the "target zone." Many heart experts feel that going over this target zone will not offer any more protection for the heart and could exceed safe limits. The target zone is considered to be 60 to 80% of a person's maximum attainable heart rate. The maximum heart rate is considered to be 220 minus a person's age. For example, a 20-year-old's maximum heart rate would be 220 minus 20, or 200 beats per minute; a 40-year-old's would be 180 beats per minute (220 minus 40), and so on. The target zone for a 20-year-old would therefore be 120 to 160 beats per minute (60 to 80% of a maximum attainable heart rate of 200); for a 40-year-old it would be 108 to 144 beats per minute.

THE HEART RATE TARGET ZONE		
Age	60%	80%
20	120	160
30	114	152
40	108	144
50	102	140
60	96	128
70	90	120

Remember that attaining your target zone and keeping it there for 20 to 40 minutes should provide all the exercise you need to get in good cardiovascular shape. There is no need to exceed these limits. When you're in the target zone, you're doing aerobic exercise and the heart and lungs are working to provide oxygen to the tissues. Beyond this, the heart and lungs can't provide enough oxygen, and anaerobia (lack of oxygen) results. Anaerobic exercise is particularly detrimental if it is prolonged, as it may cause acid toxins to develop.

Each individual reaches the target zone by different work loads. One man may attain it by just a brisk walk, another by a good jog. Age, physical conditioning, the health of the exerciser, and medications may all affect the heart rate. For anyone not in the medical field, I recommend that a physician give you some instruction on the type of exercise you should do and its duration and frequency to get you into your target zone. With this knowledge, you can modify the type of exercise you do so that you don't go over your safety limits.

June and Barbara: As June learned the hard way when she had to have injections of cortisone (a steroid) for a neuroma of the foot, steroids are a particular hazard for diabetics. They can raise blood sugar—sometimes wildly and dramatically. We also know that athletes sometimes take steroids to enhance their performance. What do you think about diabetic men using them? (We think we already know the answer to this.)

Dr. Lodewick: Steroids are a great hazard. A man should consider them only when the body lacks them or for medical indications, such as when there are not enough male hormones produced because of certain conditions or congenital deficiencies. They should *not* be used merely to allow you to outdo someone else in sports, such as Ben Johnson did when he beat Carl Lewis in the 100-meter sprint in the 1988 Summer Olympics. Overuse or improper use of steroids can lead not only to worsening of diabetes but also to high blood pressure, high cholesterol, and acceleration of heart disease. I couldn't be more negative on steroid use to improve athletic prowess for anyone—and especially for diabetics.

June and Barbara: Speaking of steroids, we know a diabetic law student who comes into the SugarFree Center. He works out at a body-building gym and is magnificently muscular—more proof that diabetics can build up large muscle mass. One day he jokingly told us that, "The word around the gyms is that insulin is the best steroid." Some of the body builders have the idea that taking insulin will help them develop bigger and better muscles, and they keep begging him to get some insulin for them. Of course he won't do it.

As far as body building for diabetics is concerned, we once heard that it's very difficult for Type I diabetics to build muscle mass, yet we've had correspondence with a Type I muscle builder who became Mr. Cincinnati and was training to go on to become Mr. Ohio. We know that muscle building is not a good idea if you have high blood pressure or eye or kidney complications. But if a diabetic man is free of these health problems, can he really build up muscle mass and expect to do as well as a nondiabetic in competition? If so, do you have any tips and precautions about how to build up muscle mass?

Dr. Lodewick: A diabetic man can build muscle mass through proper use of insulin, diet, aerobic exercise, and muscle-building exercise. Many of my Type I patients have been successful body builders, but there is a limit to each individual's capacity to build muscle mass, depending on the type and number of muscle fibers you have. This is inherited. The best example I can think of is Carl Lewis, the greatest sprinter and broad jumper in the world. No one can duplicate his athletic prowess. He was born with this capacity and he developed it to the fullest. If you're interested, not in becoming a world champion, but simply in gaining strength and muscle mass for wrestling, football, basketball, or body building, remember that your success will depend on adequate insulin supply and good diabetes control.

As far as a diabetic man being able to compete as well as a nondiabetic in body building, I'll remind you again of Tim Belknap, who was Mr. Universe in 1985 (see Chapter 3, The Trencherman). Tim developed diabetes at age 14 and was a skinny 100-pound weakling, as the muscle advertisers like to put it, until he started taking care of himself with insulin and diet. One of my patients, Chris, is an avid body builder and hopes to enter competition soon. He has what women call "a stunning build." He has attained this with excellent blood sugar control combined with a very low fat, high complex carbohydrate diet and, of course, the correct amount of insulin.

It should be emphasized here—and many people don't realize this—that insulin is not only essential for diabetes and blood sugar control but also for proper muscle development and functioning. It provides nutrients needed by the muscles, including glucose, fatty acids, and amino acids. If insulin is lacking, muscles will not use the vital glucose and amino acids properly and will weaken and break down. So Type I's must have adequate insulin to allow for building muscle mass.

However, it does take more than nutrients and insulin to build up muscle mass. Testosterone, the male sex hormone, is very important for muscle hypertrophy (enlargement), as well as for giving us men other desirable and attractive qualities. That is why men, in general, have more muscle than their female counterparts. Even among men, the amount of testosterone does vary, and this may explain part of the difference in physique among men. So for the insulin-dependent diabetic man, good blood sugar control, adequate nutrients, and the male hormone his own body produces are important for muscle development. Each man produces varying quantities, which may affect muscle size.

For superior development and strength, muscles also have to be trained and worked to capacity. Since I'm not into muscle building myself, the only advice I can give is that isometric, isotonic, and isokinetic exercises are recommended for muscle building. I would refer those of you who are interested to a sports center or to Joe Weider's *Muscle and Fitness Magazine.*

June and Barbara: Maybe at this point we could add one more valid reason for keeping diabetes in control: that out-of-control diabetes can have an adverse effect on your success in whatever sport you choose to participate.

Dr. Lodewick: It certainly can. I've seen many examples of this, but I particularly remember one boy, whose story I call:

14-YEAR-OLD GOLFER HITS BALL 300 YARDS

Kenny weighed only 99 pounds. His mother, a nurse, insisted that he needed to eat 4400 calories a day. She claimed he was testing his blood sugars at home and they were normal. I knew Kenny was fudging on the truth because his glycohemoglobin tests were always sky high. My analysis of the situation was that Kenny was eating too many calories and not taking enough insulin. As a result, his blood sugars were always high, and the glucose, instead of going into his cells to promote growth and weight gain, was going down the toilet. Instead of telling Kenny that I knew he was lying about his blood sugars, I told him that his blood sugar testing meter must not be working properly. Then I appealed to his desire for athletic prowess. Kenny loved golf and could drive a ball over 200 yards. I told him that if he had his diabetes in better control, he could probably hit it over 250 yards. This finally convinced him. He followed my advice, cut his calories, raised his insulin dose, got better control, and charted his blood sugars with honest tests. As a result, he gained 30 pounds of muscle in the next six months. Now his friends report that he can drive a golf ball 300 yards! (My next goal is to work on his putting.)

Speaking of golf, I have another memorable golf anecdote at the other end of the age spectrum—a 73-year-old man.

ONE-EYED, ONE-LEGGED MAN HITS HOLE-IN-ONE

A 73-year-old patient of mine had lost an eye as a boy from a slingshot injury and had lost a leg from gangrene when he was 70. He came to me with an ulcer on his remaining foot. This had developed because the foot was swollen and rubbed against his shoe.

After I treated him successfully for heart failure, which was responsible for the swelling, his ulcer healed. He has been back on the golf course for two years now, and just the other day he had another hole-in-one, the sixth of his career.

June and Barbara: Your patient's ulcer brings to mind the blisters and other foot injuries that a diabetic man might incur in pursuit of his sport. Since the "diabetic foot," as medical texts like to put it, is a legendary source of problems, could you engage in a little preventive medicine by sharing your experience on the subject of foot care and proper shoes and socks for sportsmen?

Dr. Lodewick: Generally diabetics in good control have no foot problems related to diabetes. So picking out the right shoes, sneakers, and socks is no different than it would be for men without diabetes. I'm not an authority on the hundreds of types of shoes available that may help performance, but I'm sure that shoes can make a difference. Roger Bannister, the first man to break the four-minute mile and now a respected neurologist, was asked how so many people have since broken his record. He answered in a typically British fashion, "It must be the shoes they are wearing."

The healthy, well-controlled diabetic without complications just needs to concern himself with preventing blisters during long, vigorous events. High on my list for this purpose are the antiblister socks made by the Double Lay-R Company (1-800-392-8500; 64 West State Street, Doylestown, PA 18901). They prevent friction at pressure sites since one layer rubs against the other instead of against your foot.

If you have poor control and/or vascular or nerve damage, this is a different story. Skin changes may be present early on without being visually apparent. The skin is an important organ system involved in diabetes. It consists of three major layers, all of which can be affected by diabetes. Although skin changes may be present on the innermost layers, the outer layer, called the epidermis, may not show manifestations until much later.

Ideally, all the skin of the foot should look like a baby's skin—silky smooth and elastic. But when, because of poor diabetes control, there is poor nutrition and poor circulation to the foot's delicate and highly traumatized skin, *then* the changes do become visually apparent. Dry skin, cracking, loss of hair, fissuring, calluses, and infection (yeast, fungal, or bacterial) of the nails and between the toes can develop. Be careful using foot products that may make the skin condition worse, such as over-the-counter medicated pads, corn pads, and solutions that may remove that waxy protective material on the outer layer of the skin.

In addition, you have to take special precautions with your feet when the nerves to your foot muscles are affected. Your muscles become weakened, and the pressure at the usual pressure points becomes magnified. This is compounded by loss of sensation so that you don't feel the pain and you lose awareness of joint and position sense. This exacerbates minor problems, such as blisters and calluses. When these sensory and neurological deficits are severe, you can develop ulcerations and pronounced foot deformities. You need to use utmost care to avoid blisters, trauma, and pressure by inspecting your feet, using antiblister socks, and keeping the skin of your feet in good condition.

Even if you have these complications of neuropathy, exercise may still be beneficial. It can prevent further loss of muscle tissue and physical fitness and can keep your hands, feet, and joints from contracting. It's important to use all your muscles as best as possible. If the severest of foot complications set in, you may have to substitute arm exercise, swimming, or bicycling for walking or jogging. Above all, if you do suffer from neuropathy, be sure—and this is crucial—to inspect your feet before, during, and after exercise to look for any new swellings, redness, or ulcerations. If you find any, report them promptly to your doctor. People with complications of the nervous system may not realize it and should ask their diabetes doctor to determine whether or not it is present.

If the arteries and blood vessels of your legs are affected by diabetes, the inadequate blood flow to your leg muscles may cause you pain. Paradoxically, although exercise seems to have a beneficial effect in improving blood flow to leg muscles, once vascular disease is present, exercise will be painful and you will want to limit the amount you do. That's why it's so important to try to prevent vascular disease in the first place. You can do this with exercise and good diabetes control, as proved in a study reported in *Diabetologia* that reviewed the history of patients with diabetes of 20 to 45 years' duration. Before exercising, however, have your doctor make sure that your heart is healthy, and once you are assured of that, then do interval training (walk, rest, walk), cycling, or upper body exercise, and you will be safe from poor blood flow in your legs.

Men frequently ask if pain in the legs is caused by arterial disease. This important aspect of leg pain needs clearing up. Most of the patients who come to me complaining about cold feet, numbness, or tingling think they have poor circulation. They don't. Rather they have nerve disease (neuropathy). The way to tell the difference between blood vessel disease and nerve disease is that blood vessel disease causes discomfort *during* exercise while neuropathy causes discomfort when you are at rest.

FINAL FOOT RECOMMENDATIONS

1. See your physician to check on whether you have any complications. If you don't, wear the shoes that are best designed for the sport you are participating in. You may also want to try wearing the Double Lay-R socks that I mentioned earlier. Keeping your feet comfortable assures you a greater chance of doing well.

2. Wash your feet daily in lukewarm water and inspect them thoroughly.

3. If you do have complications, make sure to ask the doctor the extent of the complications.

4. If you have dry skin, use a lubricating product that contains no alcohol. You might consider using some of the specially formulated products of Anastasia Marie, Inc. (1-800-542-SKIN). These products were produced especially for diabetic skin and feet by its founder, Anastasia. They are rich in natural oils that supply nutrients and therapeutic properties of lubrication vital to maintaining the optimum health, beauty, and integrity of the skin. Diabetic diabetologist, Richard K. Bernstein, M.D., recommends the use of pure refined oil of mink, which is totally nontoxic and odorless and is quickly absorbed, leaving the skin with a nonoily, velvety texture. It also keeps moisture in the skin. (Available from the SugarFree Centers.)

5. If you do have significant complications, don't fear. It's better to know you do and take precautions than to ignore them and develop an ulcerated blister and possibly infections. Wear specially molded shoes and antiblister socks and consider exercises other than walking or jogging.

6. Consult a podiatrist for foot care if you don't have perfectly healthy feet.

June and Barbara: Would you say that exercise will invariably improve a man's blood sugar control?

Dr. Lodewick: All things being equal, it will. The only problem is that all things aren't always equal. Exercise in the amounts generally recommended for cardiovascular fitness (30 to 40 minutes of exercise three or four times per week) hasn't yet been demonstrated to have a dramatic effect on long-term blood sugar control in diabetics—at least, as measured by glycohemoglobin or hemoglobin A_1C levels. One reason for this surprising phenomenon is that people who exercise this much generally consume 300 to 400 extra calories per day. They probably do this for two reasons: (1) they want to keep from getting low blood sugar, and (2) they think that their exercise allows them to eat this much more. Running three to four miles may seem like a lot, but it actually burns up only 300 to 450 calories, which are easily compensated for by consuming a mere peanut butter sandwich. Eating a favorite chocolate bar or other sweetened delight may be far in excess of the calories burned in moderate exercise.

So if you're interested in weight loss and improved blood sugar control, you must be very careful with any extra calories you consume. Skip the fudge; you be the judge! Even with exercise, you still have to rely on diet and self-control.

P O S T S C R I P T

How You Play the Game

Every time we hear the word *control*, it brings to mind an analogy of control in diabetes and control in sports—in this case Dr. Lodewick's favorite sport of tennis. Ever since Bill Talbert first stepped onto the court, there has been a special relationship between diabetes and tennis. That is as it should be. Tennis is not hazardous, yet it is as challenging and exciting as any of the bone-crushing and bruise-making sports. And although tennis is not an aerobic sport in itself, it inspires you to do aerobic exercises to build up the endurance you need to make it through a rough set on a hot afternoon.

Even more important for diabetics, as Talbert says, "Tennis is a game for life." It is a game you can play and reap the benefits of virtually forever. (The King of Sweden still played tennis when he was 90!)

Not only is tennis a game *for* life, it is also a game *of* life, as Barbara's philosopher/tennis teacher, Jeanie Mullen, constantly points out. A tennis game is a slice of life, filled with the same twists of fate and demands for patience and the courage to face adversity head on. Indeed, from the little inspirational philosophies that Jeanie serves up with the ball, it's evident that tennis and the life of a diabetic have some amazing similarities. "You play the ball; don't let the ball play you" becomes "You play your diabetes; don't let your diabetes play you." Don't just stand there watching your blood glucose levels bounce around like a missed ball. Take charge. Learn the techniques for keeping your blood glucose levels normal as much of the time as possible. The diabetes ball is in your court, so play it!

Happily, Jeanie's philosophy is a forgiving one. "It doesn't matter if you win or lose a point," she says. "The important thing is to stay loose." You also have to stay loose while controlling your diabetes. If you torture yourself over every miss (and you're bound to have some misses no matter how hard you try to follow your management program), you'll only cause more problems. Remember that stress, which can result from your guilt over a diabetes miss, can further upset your diabetes control. So no matter what happens, don't panic. Relax. Stay loose. One lost point does not make or break the match. It's your consistent and overall performance that wins games—or keeps your diabetes in control.

But teacher Mullen is tough as well as forgiving. She won't tolerate sloppiness and bad form. If you accidentally score a point when you've done everything wrong, she won't congratulate you. In fact, she'll yell at you because she doesn't want you to develop bad habits.

Someone (perhaps yourself) should yell at you if you show bad form with diabetes self-care and get away with it. For instance, if you eat a doughnut with chocolate frosting and your blood sugar doesn't go through the roof, or if you forget to eat a healthy snack and yet manage to avoid hypoglycemia, you're not to be congratulated. You are starting to develop bad habits, which are all too easy to develop. Those bad habits will eventually get you in trouble as sure as John McEnroe's mouth gets him in trouble.

According to Jeanie, after you master the basic skills, tennis is at least 50% mental control. So is diabetes. Your mental attitude is what makes you a consistent winner—or loser. Do you accept and play by the rules of the game? Do you recognize your own limitations and know how to compensate for them? Do you stay optimistic and keep your sense of humor? And above all, are you having fun? To quote Jeanie, "If you aren't having any fun, what's the point of tennis?" Or for that matter, what's the point of life—with or without diabetes? It shouldn't be a grim, teeth-gritting ordeal.

Here are a few more gems from philosopher Mullen: "Play your own game, not somebody else's. Learn what works for you and stick to it." And finally, her most important rule, something every diabetic should learn and remember: "Control is everything!"

The

WORKING MAN

• • • •

Diabetes Is Job One

The headline in the *Washington Post* tells the story: "Overachievers on Brink of Burnout Are Seeing the Light, Lightening Up." The author of the article, Cindy Skrzycki, informs us that the Japanese have a word for it: *karoshi*—death from overwork. Men often devote their mature lives to committing *karoshi* and are proud of it! In the corporation for which we briefly worked, the executives were constantly bringing up how many weeks, or even months, of vacation they had on the books that they had never used. The irony was that they considered themselves so indispensable that they couldn't be away from the job for even a day, but because of their workaholism, they were courting the Ultimate Dispensability.

Often, for a man, his career is the core of his life. But an emphasis on career to the exclusion of everything else can make that life rotten to the core. As Kenneth Pelletier, author of *Mind as Healer, Mind as Slayer*, puts it, "When work is the major value driving a person's life, it does result in some major problems."

The diagnosis of diabetes—or any other major chronic or life-threatening disease—can have the benefit of forcing you to realign your priorities. With intimations of mortality, you begin to wonder if those 50 or more hours a week 52 weeks a year on the job are what you want to do with however many hours and weeks you have left on the planet. Are there rewards other than financial success and career prominence that you'd prefer to pursue?

When you first become diabetic, you have no choice. You must instantly change one priority: diabetes becomes Job One. You have to first keep your diabetes in control if you want to successfully pursue any goal in life, career or otherwise. You must take the time out to exercise. You must get enough rest. You must eat a balanced diet. You must learn to control stress.

When you first start doing all this, you'll probably feel that everyone is watching you, thinking that you're slacking off or using your diabetes as an excuse to get out of work. This will mostly be in your own mind. Everyone else at work is probably so busy competing and trying to make *themselves* look good and worrying about what people think about *their* performance that they won't notice what you're doing.

But what about your boss or supervisor or whomever you report to? Will they feel they're not getting their money's worth out of you? Not if they're enlightened. Skrzycki reports that experts in workplace behavior predict that the aging of the baby boomers and the changing of their attitudes will create a workplace in which the number of hours will account for less and the amount of work accomplished for more. If you achieve a balance in your life between work and play, between relationships and intellectual pursuits, and between physical and emotional well-being, odds are that you will be far more creative and productive in the reasonable hours you work than if you continue to grind away in the old workaholic mode. Not only that, but in the long run you'll be able to put more time into your career because your years of work won't be cut short by *karoshi*. In fact, they'll be extended by what the Buddhists call *santi* (tranquility).

—June and Barbara

WHAT YOU'LL FIND HERE

DIABETES AND WORK PERFORMANCE

IRREGULAR WORKING HOURS AND SHIFTS

WORKING TWO JOBS

EMPLOYMENT DISCRIMINATION

GOVERNMENT PROTECTION

HIRING RESTRICTIONS

MILITARY SERVICE

HEALTH INSURANCE

June and Barbara: After reading the previous explanation that diabetes becomes Job One after the diagnosis and that it's difficult to be a diabetic workaholic, you may be asking yourself, "How can I make sure that diabetes doesn't interfere with my work performance?" We're sure, Dr. Lodewick, that since you've always carried a heavy work load yourself, you can put everyone's mind at ease on this issue.

Dr. Lodewick: The answer is very clear: keep your diabetes in good control. This should be obvious, but you'll notice as you read this chapter that I give many examples of men who take the chance of ignoring diabetes and suffer the predictable consequence of poor performance on the job. Poor control almost invariably catches up with you in the end, whereas good diabetes control can actually enhance and even improve your ability to function well.

Those of you who take insulin need to be especially careful to avoid insulin reactions at work. They can be extremely disruptive to the work environment and can affect your job security if repeated frequently.

June and Barbara: Perhaps we can add some realistic detail to that caution, as we have heard and read some amazing stories of strange behavior while under the influence of low blood sugar, or as the British call it, a "hypo."

We'll let the famous psychologist Albert Ellis, Ph.D., founder of Rational–Emotive Therapy and a diabetic for 33 years, describe his most memorable work-related hypos to you in his own words.

> Once, at an American Psychological Association convention, I walked around the halls of a Hilton Hotel loudly telling all who would hear what stupid idiots the convention officials were. Once I prepared to go down from my apartment on the top floor of the Institute for Rational–Emotive Therapy in New York to my second floor office to see my regular clients, not accepting the fact that it was three in the morning and that I was stark naked. Once, in deep insulin shock, I bit the ambulance driver who came to take me to Lenox Hill Hospital. I insisted that I was in great shape, though I was really acting like a maniac, and that I had no need of hospitalization. Luckily for me, the ambulance attendants disagreed.

Fortunately, Dr. Ellis is his own boss and didn't have to answer to anyone on these occasions. Below he tells his personal way of avoiding reactions and his own therapy for keeping the kind of control that has allowed him to function perfectly as president of the Institute for RET in New York and write more than 50 books and 600 journal articles on psychotherapy topics.

> All told, however, I have only had a half dozen serious hypoglycemic attacks in the 33 years that I have been a diabetic. I still eat about 12 times a day—precisely the right amount of carbohydrates, fats, and proteins. I exercise (which I dislike) moderately but regularly. I now take two shots of insulin every day. I test my blood sugar three or four times daily. I stay away from candy, cake, cookies, ice cream, and sweet desserts. I keep my blood pressure around 120 over 75, mainly by using no salt

and by eating a good deal of unsalted bread. And I rigorously pursue my other diabetic-controlling regimens.

Is all this easy for me to do? Hell, no! I find it time-consuming (especially since I have many other important things to do in life), often boring, and a general pain in the ass.

(From "Living with Diabetes" in the *Journal of Rational-Emotive and Cognitive-Behavior Therapy*, Spring, 1990, pp. 36–37, copyright by Institute for Rational-Emotive Therapy. Reprinted with permission)

We might add that Dr. Ellis uses his own rational–emotive therapy to help him maintain his diabetes therapy. If you want to learn more about his system of behavior modification, read his book *How to Stubbornly Refuse to Make Yourself Miserable About Anything—Yes, Anything!* or *A New Guide to Rational Living.*

June and Barbara: In *The Diabetic Woman* we remarked on how difficult keeping in control was for women because they had the stress of trying to juggle so many jobs simultaneously, as expressed in the old cliché "a woman's work is never done." What unique problems do men have dealing with their roles at work, in society, in their families, and so on, that make it hard for them to cope with diabetes?

Dr. Lodewick: I understand your point that, at least in the United States, a woman is faced with extra responsibilities. She may work hard to be successful in her career and to achieve satisfaction from it, as well as to augment the family income. In addition, she may want to be a devoted wife, mother, and housekeeper, working at home to help the family thrive. But I've never looked on life as divided between male and female jobs and responsibilities. Rather, I suggest that we look upon life as a 24-hour challenge, no matter if we are men or women or what kind of work or responsibilities we engage in. I agree with Dr. Lois Jovanovic-Peterson's analysis that it's a matter of the individual, whether man or woman, being able to take on life's challenges and cope with the stresses that assail everyone in today's society.

June and Barbara: We like to put a good face on all things diabetic, but there's no doubt that, as you keep emphasizing, an out-of-control diabetic may have trouble functioning well at work and could actually be dismissed because of incompetencies created by neglected diabetes. Have you seen any careers put in jeopardy because of neglected diabetes?

Dr. Lodewick: Yes. I recently received the following letter from one of my patients:

> Can poor control of diabetes have had an effect on my behavior? I have been accused of making a "sexual" remark to one of my female fellow employees, but I cannot remember making any comment.
>
> Also, before I went on insulin, I was accused of being insubordinate to my boss. Is it possible that poor control of my diabetes could affect my mood, memory, and thought processes? My boss said I was told that I should be doing certain tasks, but I don't remember being told to do them.
>
> I do feel much better since I went on insulin and would appreciate your opinion in this regard.

I found out that the "sexual" remark he made was, "You're looking great today, babe." If it was as simple as that, it sounds reasonably benign. However, in a strictly working relationship, a man should control the impulse to make such remarks, even if he thinks a woman looks good.

To the more important questions of could poor diabetes control make a man more lascivious and could this affect his memory and thought processes, the answer is a definite yes. Medical literature is strewn with articles indicating that patients with out-of-control Type II diabetes are more depressed, less motivated, and have impaired thinking processes.

This subject was discussed at the 1989 Annual American Diabetes Scientific Symposium. Patients with poor diabetes control performed at 80% capacity compared to nondiabetics in terms of learning and memory, according to a study by

Laurence Perlmutter of Tufts University. In a study of older Type II diabetics, Ami Laws, M.D., from the Stanford University School of Medicine, found that verbal learning, abstract reasoning, and complex psychomatic functioning were impaired compared to nondiabetics and that, the worse the diabetes control, the more likely the impairment was to occur.

Hundreds of my patients have reiterated the same point. I have one man who, when in his 60s, was definitely "slowing down," according to his wife and not as sharp as he had been. Soon after he came to me, I recommended a good diet, insulin, and an exercise program. Now in his early 80s, he walks several miles per day, travels, and has maintained his emotional and physical vitality. His wife now wishes he would "slow down a bit."

So I can definitely confirm that the patient who had been insubordinate to his boss was affected by his poor diabetes control. He had evidence of very poorly controlled diabetes and a chronic infection of the skin. After he started insulin therapy, his wife described her husband's change to a better mood and more energy as "like a miracle." She appreciated the flattering sexual remarks that he again began to make to her after a prolonged absence of such.

June and Barbara: We're glad you straightened him out so successfully and that his wife is so happy with him now. Have you seen even more dramatic and serious work problems that have been due to poor diabetes control? Some of our readers may be in trouble on the job and not even realize why and to what extremes neglected diabetes can bring a man in his career.

Dr. Lodewick: It still baffles me—although I know it's human nature—to see intelligent, sophisticated people risk their careers by refusing to educate themselves about their diabetes. In hundreds of instances, these people wait until they are on the verge of disaster before they are finally willing to do something about it. They cannot be told. They are creatures who must learn by their own experience. Unfortunately, with diabetes this approach can cost too much, even a career. As an example, I can cite the story of a lawyer patient of mine.

THE CASE OF THE PHILADELPHIA LAWYER

Helping attorneys in their predicaments of handling their own "cases of diabetes" has always been particularly satisfying to me. It seems ironic that people who spend so much time investigating and solving their clients' legal cases, devoting untold hours to delving into all the intricacies of the law, can have such difficulty in analyzing their own diabetes. Richard came to me in such a precarious situation that he had begun to question whether he had "chosen the wrong business"—that is, the law profession.

His story was one of putting in the usual heavy hours of work and study, passing the bar exam, and joining a prestigious Philadelphia law firm. In his mid-20s, he was diagnosed with diabetes, but he didn't want to admit that anything could possibly be wrong with him. He continued to ignore his condition, eating what he wanted (although avoiding sweets) and enjoying alcoholic beverages, especially to celebrate a hard-fought legal case. He disregarded self-testing of blood sugar and neglected to keep in contact with his physicians; he self-adjusted his insulin, even though he didn't understand how to do it properly.

He suffered about 10 unconscious insulin reactions requiring trips to the emergency room and several episodes of significant low blood sugar that made him so confused and befuddled that some of his clients had begun to wonder why they had retained him as their lawyer. At this point, his law firm demanded he seek medical evaluation and get straightened out or else be fired.

It was no wonder Richard had some major questions. In addition to whether he had chosen the right business, he wanted to know if he could do anything to avoid such bad insulin reactions. He was worried that he might have a serious insulin reaction and embarrass himself in front of a judge and jury. He also described what he called "tunnel vision" and could concentrate on only one thing at a time. During these periods of concentration, he could not be disturbed or it would cause him extreme irritation, and long hours would go by without his being aware that they had.

In eliciting his history further, I found out that he had hated diabetes since the minute he got it and didn't really want to hear anything about the subject. He had too many other important things to accomplish and didn't want to be bothered about the problems of diabetes. He admitted he was denying his condition.

To me, the answers to Richard's queries were as plain as day. What good did it do him to deny his diabetes? He had gone through all the effort of going to law school and joining a law firm because he liked it and looked to the satisfaction of helping many clients. The dilemma he was getting into was that by denying his diabetes, he was avoiding some simple measures that would help and thus he was on the verge of losing it all. This wise lawyer was being a fool. He could simply avoid all his trouble by learning to use blood sugar testing to guide his insulin dose, getting on a reasonable diet, and beginning some exercise activities.

I'm happy to report that Richard heeded my counsel, made some simple adjustments, and was able to carry on his career as a successful Philadelphia lawyer. He also found out that his tunnel vision problem completely disappeared, and in retrospect, we decided it most likely stemmed from periods of low blood sugar. Diabetes was no longer a problem for him now that he acknowledged it.

June and Barbara: We have a story that is the flip side of that one. Our diabetic friend, Bob, a New York stock trader, had been diagnosed only a few months before. He had accepted his diabetes perfectly and had read every book on diabetes in the New York Public Library. He had visited the Joslin Diabetes Center for more information and had put himself in the care of an eminent endocrinologist at his own expense, realizing that his HMO plan would not give him the education he desired. In spite of the good control he achieved, one morning his boss put him down with the worst comment he had ever heard. We taped Bob's story and now relate it to you exactly as he told it to us.

> The setting is the offices of a large New York stock trading company in the heart of Manhattan's financial district. The market has been down, way down, for several weeks. The work day has just begun.
>
> **Boss:** How do you feel today, Bob?
>
> **Bob:** Fine. I feel fine. No problems.
>
> **Boss:** Well, maybe you can put this diabetes thing behind you now and get back to work, because you haven't been making enough money lately.
>
> **Bob:** Don't blame it on my diabetes. For one thing, I haven't been away from work. I haven't taken one day off for diabetes, not one. Anyone else with a new disease would have taken many days off. If I'm not making money, it's because nobody's making money.

Bob said this incident really bothered him. It was, of course, blatantly wrong and unfair. The boss was just directing his anger over market conditions toward anything he could find—including an employee's diabetes. And we think Bob took just the right stance to defend himself against the boss's false accusation. The boss never attacked him on that front again. But this incident does illustrate perfectly the way management can twist things around and try to use diabetes to weaken a man's position.

June and Barbara: What if a job has irregular hours or night shifts? Isn't this particularly hard on a man with diabetes, especially an insulin-dependent man?

Dr. Lodewick: This is a question I can well understand, since in my career I've often worked 24-hour days, been deprived of sleep, and had irregular eating schedules. I know from experience that it can be handled! I know that for the insulin-dependent diabetic, like myself, it is crucial to understand the insulin's action and its relationship to food and physical activity. It's also mandatory to test your blood sugar regularly.

As long as you keep up your therapy in this way, irregular working hours and night shifts shouldn't bother you. You may, of course, have to make certain adjustments in insulin regimen and eating patterns to accommodate your new hours and work load. You will probably have to test more frequently when you first change your shift or hours, and you may have to work more closely with your physician on adjusting your insulin and eating schedules to your new working pattern.

I had a 54-year-old man come to me because he had taken on two jobs with irregular working hours and was having such severe insulin reactions that for three days he had had to be in the constant care of his lady friend. When I heard his story, his trouble with hypoglycemia was perfectly understandable. Harold had worked for 20 years in the publishing industry. During this period of time, he had had no major insulin reactions, had never been sick, and had helped his company stay in the black to the tune of 8 million dollars. He attributed his good diabetes control to the fact that he worked regular hours with regular times to take insulin, eat, and test his blood sugar. Then his company went bankrupt and he lost his job. To make a living, he started working two jobs, one during the day with lots of exercise and one from 11 P.M. to 7 A.M. as a gas station attendant. The arrangement wasn't as bad as it sounds because he could sleep a little on the night shift.

Besides all these changes in his work life, he made another very significant one in his diabetes therapy: he stopped testing his blood sugar because he felt he couldn't afford the test strips. I think his real mistake was to start taking extra doses of insulin according to how he felt.

In view of all this, it is understandable that Harold would lose track of what was going on with his diabetes, get completely out of control, and end up with incapacitating insulin shocks. I was easily able to explain to him how he had gotten himself into such a dire position, and we worked together on getting him back in good control so that he could handle his new working hours.

June and Barbara: Along this same line of inquiry, what do you think of diabetic men working more than one job as this man did?

Dr. Lodewick: If a man wants to work that hard and can keep his diabetes controlled, I see no detrimental effect. Some of my patients show real creativity when it comes to combining jobs. One man is a minister, and since he's married and has a young daughter, he needed a little more cash to defray expenses and the potential cost of raising and educating a child. He took on a sales job for Mobil Oil and more than tripled his income. What he had learned from his years at the pulpit about eloquent delivery helped him become quite a persuasive salesman.

June and Barbara: Can you offer some advice on career choice? In particular, which jobs are diabetic men legally prevented from holding and which would you consider inappropriate?

Dr. Lodewick: I've always thought that the ideal career for a diabetic would be a mail carrier because you get a lot of exercise and have good health benefits. But if being a swift courier through the snow and rain and heat and gloom of night doesn't have appeal for you, there is still a world of possibilities.

In choosing a career, a diabetic man has to consider the same factors that every man has to consider, but in addition he must face the reality that if he takes insulin, certain jobs are legally prohibited to him or simply not recommended. Jobs that an insulin-taking diabetic man should not hold are those in which his own welfare or the welfare and lives of others may be in jeopardy because of the possibility of hypoglycemia. The federal government does not allow diabetics on insulin to enter the armed forces, to pilot airplanes, or to drive trucks or buses in interstate commerce. Any job that involves the use of dangerous machinery, such as boat operation or crane operation, should be ruled out if you take insulin or even oral hypoglycemics.

Aside from these restrictions, I wish to emphasize that diabetes should not prevent you from a physically active job, regardless of whether you're on insulin or not. For Type II's who do not take insulin or oral hypoglycemic pills, any job choice is fine, as long as you have not developed any complications.

To give you some specific guidance, here is a short list of examples of "good" job choices and "bad" job choices. But remember, there are really as many careers open to you as your imagination allows.

Good Choices		Bad Choices
Art	Law	Fireman
Music	Baker	Policeman
Medical Fields	Clergy	Tree Trimmer
Engineering	Computers	Airplane Pilot
Journalism	Insurance	Bus Driver
Photography	Hotels	Truck Driver
Advertising	Locksmith	Roofer
Marketing	Secretary	Armed Forces
Stenography	Pharmacist	
Bookkeeping	TV–Radio	
Accounting	Dietitian	
Clerical		

This is just a small selection of jobs, but you can see that there are many more good choices than bad choices. In making these choices, many men may also want to think seriously about going for jobs that allow them to get good medical and life insurance coverage.

Incidentally, one of my patients, a very enterprising businessman, got himself into a career that you might think would be totally inappropriate for a diabetic. He was originally part owner of a gasoline station franchise, when the oil crunch of the late 1970s caused his parent oil company to deprive him of his usual profit. Jolted by this turn of events, he quickly saw another business opportunity—starting a fancy candy store. You might think it ironic that a diabetic would run a candy store, but who would know sweets better? There are even some sweets made with fructose or mannitol that may not cause as much metabolic effect on blood sugar or blood fats. (These are available at the SugarFree Centers.)

If you are at a loss for help in employment counseling, go to the Department of Vocational Rehabilitation in your state. They can help you find careers or assign you a trained counselor who will obtain funds for you to receive psychological or social counseling or on-the-job training, if such funds are available.

June and Barbara: We've heard of many cases of discrimination against diabetics in the employment market. We'd like to know of experiences with discrimination your patients have had in the workplace and if you have been able to help them in any way.

Dr. Lodewick: Discrimination can be a major obstruction to finding a good job, as many of my patients have unfortunately encountered. In fact, I've seen some of my young aspiring patients even turned down for medical school because someone on the admission committee considered a career in medicine too stressful for a person with diabetes. Those of you who have doctors with diabetes know what a mistake this is. As one diabetic patient put it, "A diabetic doctor is a good combination from the patient's standpoint. Diabetes is a subjective condition, and one has to be diabetic to really understand and appreciate it."

This is certainly not to say that all people with diabetes should be doctors! There is a great deal of stress and long hours in this profession. As I mentioned earlier, Elliott Joslin, considered to be the pioneer in education and self-management of diabetes and the founder of the world-renowned Joslin Center in Boston, often recommended that people with diabetes should not aspire to be number one, but should settle for being second best to relieve themselves of stress. So rather than becoming physicians, many people who are oriented to the health field might consider nursing, psychology, social work, anesthesia, or hospital or health-care management. There is much satisfaction and reward in helping people in this field with somewhat less stress. For those who want to be doctors, some of the less stressful specialties, such as dermatology or radiology, provide rewarding pursuits without the stress that surgery and other specialties may carry.

To return to the subject of discrimination, it was reported in the December 1989 issue of *Diabetes Forecast* that Carolyn Willard was turned down for a job because of diabetes. According to the story, she applied for a job selling health, life, and accident insurance. She took the prerequisite examination and scored the highest of any applicant. Despite this and her otherwise excellent background, the employer of the firm denied her the job because he considered it "too stressful for a person with diabetes."

Besides Carolyn, many other people with diabetes have been denied work or job opportunities or, even worse, lost jobs because of such discrimination. Many employers no doubt base their decisions on ignorance, not knowing that some of the greatest people alive have diabetes and it has not affected their performance. Other employers may have other reasons for not hiring a person with diabetes, for equally invalid reasons. Because of this, it has been necessary for many diabetics not to inform their employers or prospective employers that they have diabetes. I know many people in this category.

At this point I have two stories to illustrate that you can fight this discrimination and win.

MAN FOOLS A MAJOR DRUG CONGLOMERATE

Though Stanley had had diabetes since he was a youth, he had a fine job working for a large drug conglomerate. After working effectively there for over 10 years and assuming a major position with the company, he, like many of us men, looked for even greener pastures. Offered a high-paying job by another drug conglomerate, he made a major mistake. He gave up his first job before being hired for the second, not knowing that he would have to pass a physical examination with the new firm. As bad luck would have it, he came down with a very curious medical condition called sarcoidosis—a condition unconnected with diabetes that affects the lungs, liver, and skin. The new company would not hire him unless he could prove that this condition was under control. He had wisely not informed them that he also had diabetes, which would have meant double trouble.

We worked on controlling both his sarcoidosis and his diabetes. When Stanley had his physical examination, he had normal blood sugar, and there was nothing to indicate diabetes. He passed his examination and got the job.

MAN BEATS THE IRS

In this instance, Tom, a 25-year-old man, came down with diabetes and was placed on insulin just as he was expecting a major promotion in the security division of the Internal Revenue Service. The Internal Revenue, for whatever reason, would not give Tom the promotion unless he could prove that he didn't need insulin. He went to two doctors, but they concluded that he was insulin-dependent. When I saw him six months after his diabetes was diagnosed, it was my analysis that he was getting reasonable blood sugar control on only 16 units of insulin, but that he was 15 pounds overweight. In addition, he was on a 2500-calorie diet and consuming eight ounces of orange juice and one quart of milk daily. (I find too many calories are often prescribed to diabetic patients.) After he eliminated the milk and orange juice and added exercise, he was able to stop taking insulin and his blood sugars remained normal. I wrote a letter to his employer indicating that he no longer needed insulin and that there was no sign of diabetes. He got his deserved promotion.

Tom was fortunate that he could go off insulin. Had he been a Type I diabetic who had to take it, he would not have been able to get the promotion. But in cases such as Tom's, it is always wise to consult with a diabetes specialist who may be able to solve the problem or, failing that, to try to work with the company to educate them as to how a diabetic on insulin can actually handle the job with no problems.

June and Barbara: We recently read about a man who lost his job because of his diabetes—or so he claimed. Bruce Trow was a stockbroker working for an office of Dean Witter–Reynolds in Florida. He had been hired in 1985, a year after being diagnosed diabetic. He told his employers about his diabetes when he was hired and said that it never seemed to be an issue with them. In 1987, Trow developed high blood pressure and was advised by a psychologist that job stress might be aggravating his condition.

As a result of this diagnosis, Trow took a two-week medical leave in January 1988. On February 15, he told his employer that he planned to file for disability benefits and take a long-term leave. On February 25 when Trow asked the branch manager about the progress of the paperwork on his disability claim, he was told that he was being terminated on February 25 because his production was declining.

After investigating the case, the Florida Commission on Human Relations ruled that since Trow was one of the top-performing account executives in the office, the claim of poor sales performance was just an excuse for the dismissal and that the state's antidiscrimination law likely had been violated. The commission investigator stated that Trow's firing was "particularly suspect because it happened just after he had notified the company of his intention to seek disability benefits" and thus there was reasonable cause to believe that Dean Witter–Reynolds had discriminated against Trow because of his diabetes.

As in any dispute of this sort, the waters were muddied with claims and counterclaims on both sides. The company said that they employed many diabetics—there was even one in the same office as Trow—and that diabetes was never a criterion either for hiring or dismissal. They cited a number of purely business reasons for Trow's dismissal and appealed to the commission to reconsider their decision. But before the commission could act on the request, Trow filed a civil lawsuit against Dean Witter–Reynolds and the branch manager, seeking back pay and an unspecified amount of compensatory and punitive damages.

Trow maintains that "since this happened to me, I haven't slept well. I have nightmares about it, and my blood sugar and blood pressure readings are all out of whack. But if this can help some other diabetic facing a situation like mine, then it's worth it." It will be interesting to see how this case turns out. It may establish a precedent that will influence future discrimination against diabetics in the job market for better or worse.

Do you know of any other clear-cut cases in which a diabetic man was actually fired from his job because of discrimination?

Dr. Lodewick: The case I know of was probably not actual discrimination, but the man did get fired. The problem was that he developed diabetes *after* holding the job for a number of years. If he had been diabetic at the onset, he would not have been hired for such dangerous work and the employer could not have been accused of discrimination for refusing to employ him.

This man was a very loyal, dedicated hard worker who put in long hours and was rarely sick or absent from work, even though he did important shift work driving a forklift. When he developed diabetes in his early 40s, he continued to feel well over the next 10 years. He followed the advice of his physician and took on the responsibility of learning as much as possible about the details of treatment. He even observed, to his dismay, that some of his fellow employees were sick and did sloppy work as a consequence of overindulging in alcohol and drugs. He was proud that he could carry on his duties despite having diabetes.

But then he began having trouble with sleepiness, confusion, and bursts of temper that came on intermittently. These spells were brought on by low blood sugar reactions. His company felt that these types of reactions were too dangerous, and they placed him on disability. He was understandably angered. Why should he lose his job, when he had never missed a day's work, while some of his co-workers were frequently sick or abused alcohol or drugs and even had accidents on the job? They were allowed to continue working. It definitely seemed unfair.

He did admit that he had "rare low blood sugar reactions" at work. But he felt he could prevent them in the future. He also argued that other men performing the same job might have a heart attack or an alcohol incident and yet they weren't put on disability. He sought my opinion.

Initially I empathized with his position. I thought that with frequent self-testing of blood sugar every two or three hours and proper snacking he could maintain his blood sugar above 100 mg/dl and thus avoid insulin reactions. I even wrote a letter to his company physician explaining this. But he replied that, despite my expertise in diabetes, he thought I should observe the working conditions of this man to better formulate an opinion. It was true that I was not familiar with the internal operations of his company, having never seen the actual working environment firsthand. The company physician invited me down to visit the plant.

After my visit, I knew this man was not being discriminated against. His job was dangerous. He drove the forklift down very narrow pathways carrying 1000-pound bales, which could tumble over him or others or down a subway pier, if he should get significantly confused from hypoglycemia. I recommended that, because of the many good years this man had put in at the company, they consider finding him a more suitable and less dangerous position. Unfortunately, there were no such jobs available with the company, so he had to seek employment elsewhere.

June and Barbara: Let's assume that a diabetic man has a genuine case of job discrimination to fight. What protection does the government provide for diabetics in such circumstances?

Dr. Lodewick: A special President's Committee on the Employment of the Handicapped, which includes diabetics, was formed in the 1980s. The mission of this committee is "to encourage employers, the medical profession, and other interested parties to adopt and utilize practices that will facilitate the hiring and progression in employment of qualified handicapped individuals." There is a special report from this committee that includes medical expert advice on the employment of people with diabetes. Here are the stipulations of this report.

1. Well-controlled, properly supervised, cooperative diabetics without serious complications are "good risk" employees capable of safe and efficient service in appropriate jobs for which they are vocationally qualified.

2. Federal regulations, as well as many state and local laws, have made it illegal for most employers to reject an applicant on the basis of the disease alone. As long as

they can perform the work and *present no hazard to themselves or others, they cannot be denied employment.*

3. Both the employee and the employer should cooperate to monitor diabetic employees, assist them to adjust to the workplace, and place restrictions on their activities as necessary.

4. It may be out of bounds to require an employee who does not seem to be having any work-related problems to undergo periodic medical exams.

5. Employees should educate all personnel department staff and supervisory personnel on diabetes and make them aware of emergencies and how they should be handled.

6. Personnel and medical staff should confer with diabetic employees on any ways that they can accommodate one another to prevent work-related or medical problems.

A federal agency called the Office of Personnel Management has been created to look into the safety aspects of various jobs for the handicapped. (You can find its telephone number in the white pages under United States Government Offices, Office of Personnel Management.) This office has delineated two categories of jobs: nonhazardous and hazardous. In non-hazardous positions, no restrictions are placed on employees, except that some consideration must be given for positions that entail irregular hours or are located in geographical areas where there is limited medical care available. Hazardous positions are those in which a diabetic could be at additional risk if he or she had a diabetes complication affecting the heart, vision, or neurological system or had had serious hypoglycemic reactions in the previous year.

This shows why it is crucially important for you to take good care to prevent medical complications. I can't reiterate too often the importance of not ignoring your diabetes even though you feel well. Do not assume that feeling well proves that you are in control and are preventing complications. You must be practicing good self-treatment and have good blood sugars to verify it.

June and Barbara: In light of these restrictions on hiring men with diabetes, what actually happens when a diabetic man goes to a company to apply for a position? What is the screening process like?

Dr. Lodewick: It often depends on whether you're dealing with a small company or a large corporation. In a small company, the personnel manager is often the one to decide whether to hire or not. There is the danger that the manager, not knowing enough about diabetes, may permit a diabetic man taking insulin and prone to hypoglycemia to assume a position that he is ill-suited for, such as one involving the use of dangerous equipment or working on scaffolding. This may also happen if the prospective employee's own physician is used to help determine if the job is appropriate for him. The personal physician is biased toward his patient and doesn't have the needed familiarity with the operation of the company and its internal environment. And the patient, anxious to secure the job and confident he can take on all the requirements, does not inform his personal physician of all the details of the working environment for fear the physician may not recommend him.

In a large company, approval for employment must come from the company physician. One case I heard of involved a young diabetic man who, after graduating and receiving his M.B.A. degree, went for an introductory job interview with a major drug company that manufactures an oral hypoglycemic and is well known for its diabetes education program. This company was enthusiastic about hiring this young man for a sales position. All he needed to do was pass the medical examination. When the company physician found out he had diabetes, he recommended that the man not be hired, pointing out that diabetes *might* cause a number of medical problems for the applicant *in the future*, even though it had caused him no difficulties up to then, he had no complications, and his control was good.

When personnel management heard this, they were understandably upset. As one of the marketing managers related, "That's like saying no one should be employed after age 55 because he might have a heart attack."

The personnel department overturned the physician's recommendation and hired the young man anyway. The decision so far has been a very good one, as he's been one of the most productive salesmen on their sales force. In the meantime, the company physician has been updated and enlightened on diabetes.

Another problem with larger companies is that the company physician may be leery of recommending employment that requires physically active work for an insulin-dependent diabetic. Some of these physicians may just be overly cautious and conservative. They may feel that if they *never* recommend that a diabetic be allowed to work on a ladder or with dangerous equipment, then they will not have to worry about diabetics who get injured on the job. Also, they will not have to worry about malpractice suits from injured employees, if this should indeed occur.

It is important for employers and employees to have as much knowledge about diabetes as possible so as to not unnecessarily limit the employability of a diabetic in even a very physically demanding position. Again, I must emphasize that diabetes per se need not limit a man from a very physically active job, regardless of whether the diabetic takes insulin or not. Employers must be made knowledgeable in this respect. Remind them of such men as Carl Johnson, who although diabetic since the age of 14, has performed the iron man triathlon (2-mile swim, 26-mile run, and 125-mile bike ride), and of many other athletes with diabetes. However, the employee himself should attempt to avoid chronically poor blood sugar control and so offset or prevent the medical complications of diabetes that may also result in loss of work. And the employer should be eager to work with the diabetic employee and his physician to enable him to serve his company best.

June and Barbara: We are sure you'll agree that many discriminatory practices of the past will no longer be possible since the Americans with Disabilities Act was signed into law by President Bush in July 1990. Under this law, diabetes is legally considered a disability. It is termed a *hidden disability* along with heart disease, cancer, and epilepsy. So now if you work for a private employer who has 15 or more employees and you feel you have been discriminated against, you can file a complaint and have the situation corrected if you can show you are a "qualified individual." *Qualified* here means you can perform the essential functions of the job.

Under this law, employers also have to make "reasonable accommodation" for a person's health needs. So you have a right to ask for work or lunch hours that will make it possible for you to take time for insulin injections, blood sugar testing, and visits to your doctor.

This is a good place for us to mention that not all employers have to be forced to accommodate the needs of diabetics. Some go out of their way to be understanding and supportive. In the Summer 1990 issue of *Countdown*, the magazine of the Juvenile Diabetes Foundation International, we read the story of what the U.S. Balloon Manufacturing Company did to accommodate the handicap of 66-year-old Marion Gerard, a diabetic for 25 years, who while in their employ had had both legs amputated. Marion, we should point out, "is perhaps the company's best sales representative," and when the company moved to a new part of Brooklyn quite a distance from her home, they literally took her with them. The company provides ambulette service to take Marion to and from work, a motorized vehicle that enables her to get around the office, and a wheelchair and walker. In addition, they are looking into getting her a special computer, because she is beginning to have vision problems. And although U.S. Balloon has a group health insurance plan, the company was unable to get Marion into it, so the company arranged a personal comprehensive policy for Marion with no deductible.

A final plus of the Americans with Disabilities Act is that it restricts employers from asking you whether you have diabetes. They can still ask *after* they have given you a conditional offer of employment, but only if they need to know for safety reasons. So things are really looking up.

June and Barbara: What about jobs in the military? Are they absolutely inflexible about letting diabetics join? No exceptions? We know one young diabetic man whose life dream was to join the U.S. Marine Corps. This dream was shattered when he was turned down flat and told that he could never be a Marine because of his diabetes. This kind of exclusionary rule smacks of discrimination in its most virulent form. You'd think a government agency could do a little better in treating all its citizens fairly. What happens if you are already in the armed forces when diagnosed?

Dr. Lodewick: As I said in my introduction, I was serving in the Navy as a doctor in 1968 when first diagnosed and I suffered the injustice of not being allowed to continue. The U.S. Naval Medical Officer responsible for this decision indicated that it was Navy regulations that all military persons have to be ready to go anywhere, anytime, in case of a war emergency. No matter how hard I insisted that as a doctor I could serve in a non-war zone, it was to no avail. U.S. military regulations forbade it and there was nothing I could do about it.

Before 1969, any serviceman developing diabetes requiring insulin, even top-ranked officers near retirement, could no longer serve. Since then, there have been some changes in regulations so that in exceptional cases, they will keep some insulin-dependent diabetics who are already in. Generally, Type II non-insulin-dependent men who are career military personnel will be kept in the service even if they develop their diabetes while on active duty. However, neither Type II's nor Type I's are allowed to join the service.

Finally, to show how tough and unfair military regulations are, I can also give my son Matt's experience. Matt was ecstatic when he received word that he had been awarded a Navy ROTC scholarship to college. It pended, however, on his passing the physical examination. Since he enjoys good health, he thought he would pass easily. He was greatly disappointed when he was turned down because he is colorblind. Why being colorblind should make anyone unfit to be in the Navy in today's world is incredible to me, but it demonstrates the inflexibility of military regulations.

June and Barbara: The one small sliver of a silver lining in the cloud of military service for diabetics is that if you develop Type I diabetes while in the service, you get a lifetime disability pension, which can be as high as 80%. We have one friend who was diagnosed in his early 20s when he was in the Navy and has been receiving a pension ever since, and he's now about 60.

Pat Ockel, the manager of our Del Mar SugarFree Center, was formerly in the Navy medical corps. When her diabetes was diagnosed she was no longer on active duty so she couldn't get a pension (even though she was a member of the reserves). Ironically, if her diabetes had been diagnosed during her annual two weeks of active duty, she would have been eligible for one!

Pat says she suspects that there are quite a few diabetic Chiefs in the Navy. She says when she was in the service, the joke was that you had to have a beer gut to make Chief. When being overweight combines with the added years, it stands to reason that a number of cases of diabetes are likely to appear. She figures that many of these men—even if they really need insulin—stay on pills so they can remain in the service. The result of this would be poor diabetes control, which could diminish the number of years they would be able to enjoy their pensions when they eventually did retire.

Dr. Lodewick: Pat is certainly right about that. Incidentally, one good feature about retiring from the military, whether after the full 20 years or less as a result of diabetes, is that both the man and his family are then entitled to military medical care.

June and Barbara: That is indeed an advantage. Getting good medical insurance if you have diabetes has become a formidable challenge. We recently heard a health insurance commercial on the radio in which two managers were talking about trying to hire a hot-shot employee. They worried they were going to lose him to the competition which had a better health insurance plan. The solution in the commercial, of course, was for the company to sign on with the better insurance company themselves. Exaggerated though this may be, it did point out how important health insurance is becoming. If you are looking for a job—especially if you have a chronic disease such as diabetes—you should thoroughly investigate a firm's health insurance plan before signing on.

Even if you join a company that has excellent health insurance, in some cases a "preexisting condition" such as your diabetes won't be covered for a certain period. That period can be as long as 24 months. However, if a company really wants you, you can probably negotiate a deal to have the company pay the doctor and supply costs of taking care of your preexisting condition until the insurance kicks in. For a Type I man that could run as much as $200 a month.

Then there's the government's COBRA plan. COBRA is an acronym for the government act that brought it into being: the Consolidated Omnibus Budget Reconciliation Act of 1986. The COBRA strikes if you quit or are terminated by an employer that has 20 or more employees. What it does is give you the right to continue the insurance you had with your former employer for a period of up to 18 months. Unfortunately, you have to pay the premium. Fortunately, should you have an accident or develop a new health problem (if that can be considered fortunate!), the insurance company is obliged to keep you covered until the condition is alleviated, even if that takes far longer than

18 months. When you get insurance from the next company you go to work for, then you're no longer eligible for COBRA. It's only for people who have no other health insurance.

If you are in business for yourself, you already know how virtually impossible it is for an individual to afford private health insurance—even if that individual doesn't have diabetes or any other chronic condition. If you're not in business for yourself, but are considering doing it, be sure to look into insurance coverage problems before you leap. Unless your wife has family coverage where she works, it may not be financially feasible for you to strike out on your own at this time.

We say *at this time* because there are heavy rumblings of discontent being heard across the land. If some type of federal health insurance plan isn't enacted to make affordable health care accessible to everyone—with or without chronic diseases—a number of politicians are likely to lose their sinecures. You might tell them so. That kind of threat prods politicians into action when nothing else will. We have strong hopes, therefore, that it won't be long before you no longer have to let your career choice be influenced by the health plan it provides.

There's already help available if you live in Connecticut, Florida, Georgia, Illinois, Indiana, Iowa, Maine, Minnesota, Montana, Nebraska, New Mexico, North Dakota, Oregon, South Carolina, Tennessee, Texas, Washington (State), or Wisconsin. These states have pooled risk insurance. This means that any insurance company doing business in that state must contribute to a fund that makes health insurance available to people who would otherwise not be able to get health insurance at all or would be able to get it only at impossibly exorbitant rates. The maximum that they can charge for such insurance is 125 to 150% of the average premium in that particular state. If you live in a pooled risk state, any well-informed insurance agent should be able to tell you how to get onto this plan.

As far as automobile and life insurance are concerned, the problems are much less significant. In fact they're virtually non-existent. Some automobile insurance companies don't even ask if you're diabetic. If they do ask and you tell them—as, of course, you must or risk invalidating the policy—about all they generally require is a doctor's letter saying that you're in good control. Those reasons for keeping yourself in good control just keep adding up.

If the company you work for provides all employees with a life insurance policy, you'll almost always be covered just like everybody else. For individual policies, if you take fewer than 40 units of insulin or none at all and, here we go again, *you are in good control*, you can get a policy as easily as a nondiabetic.

POSTSCRIPT

Putting Out Fires Without Getting Burned

Before we leave the workplace, we have one more message for you. Although diabetes is Job One and without first handling it well, you can't do Job Two, it's a mistake to become obsessive and rigid about your self-care regimen. We have seen some prime examples of this at the SugarFree Centers. All things being equal, we go out of our way to hire diabetics since they bring a special understanding to their jobs. Sometimes June at our Van Nuys Center or Pat at our Del Mar Center will have to pop a few Dextrosols and delay lunch or a snack until a client who really needs their special help can be taken care of. And yet we've had other employees who were so wrapped up in their own diabetes that no one else's needs seemed of importance to them.

One young man worked for us part-time from 9 A.M. to 1:30 P.M. because he was pursuing an acting career and wanted his afternoons free for auditions. Despite the fact that it made our scheduling extremely difficult, he insisted on eating his lunch precisely at 12:30—no variations, *ever*—because that was when he "had to eat" for his diabetes control. This meant he took his half-hour lunch and then came back to work for only a half hour. The strange thing was that we never saw him take his blood sugar to see if he was really low and really had to eat at that exact moment.

Then we had another employee with just the opposite problem. He didn't want to be scheduled for a definite lunch hour because he never knew when he might need to eat. It could be as early as 11:00 A.M. or as late as 2:00 P.M., depending on his blood sugar vagaries of the day. Again, the scheduling became a heavy problem since his co-workers never knew when he might want to eat. When he did, they were expected to drop their own work instantly and cover for him.

Since we are totally involved with diabetes care, we were accommodating to a fault. But it seems unlikely that most businesses and co-workers would be able or willing to make the adjustments we did. And in most cases, it shouldn't even be necessary. There are many ways to adjust insulin schedules and eating patterns to fit your particular work situation and still give you optimum diabetes control.

Then there is the other problem associated with rigid fixation on your diabetes control. What do you do when there's a huge job crisis that you absolutely have to handle? We think you should follow the advice of Dr. Lois Jovanovic-Peterson. In *The Diabetic Woman* she maintains that "when something really traumatic happens. . . it is normal to forget diabetes self-care. . . . It is best to cope with the disaster and avoid feeling guilty about transient loss of diabetes control. Then, when the crisis has passed, diabetes control can take center stage again."

Strangely enough, Dr. Jovanovic-Peterson recently experienced just such a situation herself on the homefront, but it's a good example of what you might experience on the workfront. She and her husband, Charles Peterson, M.D., another diabetes specialist, live with their family of teenagers in a canyon area of Santa Barbara, California. On this particular evening Lois was fixing dinner and her husband was watching the evening news on TV. The announcer was telling about the fire that was roaring down San Antonio Creek Canyon, the very canyon in which they live. Charles looked out the window and THERE IT WAS roaring straight at their house! He shouted to the family and they all went out and started hosing down the roof and the foliage. Lois, of course, went with them.

The family worked together for hours fighting the fire. In the back of her mind, Lois undoubtedly realized that she hadn't taken her predinner insulin and that adrenaline, activated by the situation, was probably shooting her blood sugar into the stratosphere. She finally ran inside when there was a momentary break in the fire's intensity and without checking her blood sugar or even measuring the insulin, drew up a big dose, shot it in, and raced back to fight the fire. Was her diabetes out of control during this period? Absolutely! Should she have said to her husband, ''Chuck, you and the kids go out and fight the fire. I have to test my blood sugar and take my insulin and eat dinner. I'll see you later when I've finished''? Absolutely not!!

So when your job hands you a major crisis, do what you must do to get through it, even if your diabetes has to take a temporary back seat. And do it with a clear conscience—stewing over it only makes the situation worse. If, however, you find that every day at work is nothing but constant crises, that all you do is put out fires, then it may be time to think seriously about getting a different Job Two. After all, you don't want to jeopardize your lifetime contract with Job One.

The
SEXUAL MAN
· · · ·
A Potent Argument for Good Diabetes Control

One day we were talking to diabetic comedian Tom Parks, who told us that he was trying to work up a diabetes segment for his comedy act. It went something like this:

This guy was in his doctor's office to get the results of a physical. The doctor delivered to him the news that the diagnosis was diabetes. Like most people, the guy knew nothing about diabetes.

"What does this mean, Doc? What's going to happen to me?"

"Well," said the doctor, "if you don't take care of yourself, it could cause kidney failure and you'd have to go on dialysis."

"Gee, Doc, that's pretty rough, but if it happens, it happens and I'll handle it. Is there anything else?"

"You could get an infection and have to have a foot or even a leg amputated."

"Wow! It's that bad?! I didn't realize. But I'll be a man about it. I can live with it. Is there more that can happen?"

"Yes. Diabetes is one of the leading causes of blindness."

"*Blindness*?!! That's terrible. Blindness! It won't be easy, but I'll manage if I have to. Is that all?"

197

"Not quite. Uncontrolled diabetes frequently causes impotence."

"*WHAT!* NO!! NOT THAT!!! I CAN'T TAKE IT!!!! SAY IT ISN'T SO!!!! ANYTHING BUT THAT!!!!!! I'D RATHER DIE."

Tom hadn't worked out the whole segment then. Maybe he's still putting it together. Then again, maybe he gave up the idea because, in reality, diabetic impotence is no laughing matter. Diabetes health professionals report that many men have a similar reaction to the one in Tom's routine.

Sex, after all, is a major aspect of a man's life. Dr. Keren Shaynor in *The Shaynor Study: The Sexual Sensitivity of the American Male* reports that men between the ages of 12 and 40 think of sex on an average of six times per hour. The way this breaks down is that between the ages of 12 and 19, it's 20 times per hour, and between the ages of 30 and 39, it diminishes to a mere four times per hour. With this much focus on sex, it isn't surprising that diabetic men regard impotence as a major concern of their disease, if not *the* major concern. In fact, when we asked in the *Health-O-Gram* for questions that diabetic men would like answered, there were three times as many questions on sex as on any other topic.

It's not surprising, then, that impotence looms as the number one concern of diabetic men. Our goal for this section of the book is to put your fears on this topic to bed, or at least into perspective.

—June and Barbara

WHAT YOU'LL FIND HERE

IMPOTENCE

ROLE OF HORMONES, VASCULAR SYSTEM, AND NERVOUS SYSTEM

MEDICAL EVALUATION AND TESTS

SELF-HELP ORGANIZATIONS

DIABETES CONTROL AND IMPOTENCE

PSYCHOLOGICAL FACTORS

PSYCHOLOGICAL COUNSELING

PHYSICAL FACTORS

VACUUM ENTRAPMENT DEVICES

NONENTRAPMENT DEVICES

MEDICATIONS

PENILE IMPLANTS

SEX THERAPY

VASECTOMY

STERILITY

June and Barbara: Does impotence loom as the horrifying spectre in a man's life that Tom Parks portrays it?

Dr. Lodewick: Definitely! Impotence is one of the greatest fears a man has. Many men say, "The day it does not go up is the day I want to die." It can be a heartbreaking experience, especially when "the mood is there but the car won't go," as one of my patients described his frustrating predicament.

Impotence is tied up with complex emotions. It can give a man a feeling of inadequacy and loss of masculinity. It can attack and undermine his self-esteem. Just as women like to be told that they're beautiful, men like to think of themselves as handsome or attractive, and loss of sexual functioning can be a definite downer to this feeling.

The desire to relate to a person of the opposite sex starts early in a boy's development. As soon as the male hormone, testosterone, begins exerting its effect on the growing adolescent, a boy begins to see his female counterpart as beautiful for the first time and tries to engage her in some kind of sexual encounter. He revels in his successful experiences (which do not have to be intercourse, but just the realization that he is ready and able should the situation present itself) and acknowledges this to his male friends. As he matures, he sees that there is much more involved in a meaningful man–woman relationship than strictly a sexual one and will become interested in these other aspects as well. However, he may still feel that a sexual encounter is absolutely necessary to react comfortably with a woman. The loss of sexual ability can be a severe blow to him; he certainly wants to give his female partner satisfaction in their sexual relationship. This is where impotence can be a problem, and impotence is quite common with diabetes.

June and Barbara: Just how widespread is impotence in the male population in general and in diabetic men specifically?

Dr. Lodewick: More common than most people realize. There may be as many as 15 million men in the United States affected by it. When there's not a psychological cause, diabetes is the most common reason for impotence. In varying studies, up to 50% of diabetic men over the age of 50 have some degree of impotence. Even in diabetic men under 30 years of age, 15 to 20% may be impotent.

Impotence is sometimes the initial manifestation of diabetes. In a study reported in the *Journal of the American Medical Association*, a group of 63 men with normal sexual function was compared to a group of 55 men with impotence. Twelve percent of the impotent men had abnormal blood sugars, whereas no cases of glucose intolerance occurred in the group of men with normal sexual functioning.

June and Barbara: Is there a difference in the incidence of impotency between Type I and Type II diabetics?

Dr. Lodewick: Because there are many more men with Type II diabetes, Type II's have the greater incidence of impotency. In fact, because Type II diabetes is so subtle and may not have any disturbing symptoms, it can linger on uncontrolled for a number of months or years before it is finally diagnosed. If a man feels well, he will be less likely to seek medical attention until a complication such as impotence finally develops.

Type I men are more aware of their diabetes at an earlier onset. They may do more to keep it controlled and, therefore, prevent the complication of impotence from ever developing. Far more men suffer impotence if their diabetes has been poorly controlled compared to those who have been well controlled.

And for the benefit of you curious readers interested in knowing my own status, I can reassure you that, despite over 20 years of diabetes and at the age of 49, I enthusiastically support a good sexual drive and my sexual ability remains as good as it was in my raw youth, although the years have made me a much better lover (at least, I hope Maureen thinks so!).

June and Barbara: There is so much misunderstanding about impotence that it would help if you could define the term so we all have the same information base to work from.

Dr. Lodewick: Impotence means the inability to have a firm enough erection sufficient for penetration and completion of the sexual act. Often impotence is coupled with normal libido and ability to ejaculate, which makes it particularly frustrating. To have an erection, men need their minds and bodies to cooperate. Erection is a complex process involving psychological, endocrine, vascular, and neurological systems.

June and Barbara: Let's take these systems one at a time so we can find out the part each plays and what problems could exist with each. The psychological part is the one that makes us afraid to even talk about impotence. Many diabetic men are doing just fine until they read or hear that diabetes can cause impotence, and then instant impotence can develop, which may take extensive psychological counseling to work out. Men who become nervous and anxious about the possibility of impotence may start observing and monitoring their sexual experiences, "spectatoring" as it's called in sexual therapy circles. This can diminish both pleasure and performance. Let's hope that you diabetic men who have no sexual problems (except for the occasional ones that all men have) keep it that way and don't start worrying about impotence. In fact, you might want to skip the next three questions and answers lest they make you try to fix something that ain't broke. But for those of you who feel you have some emerging problem or just have intellectual curiosity on the subject, let's proceed by first looking at the endocrine system. What part do hormones play?

Dr. Lodewick: Just as insulin is a hormone that controls blood sugar and other substances needed for growth and development, there are many hormones that control sexual functioning. At least three hormones produced by the brain affect the proper functioning of the testes and cause the production of the male hormone testosterone and/or the production of sperm: gonadotropin-releasing hormone (GRH), luteinizing hormone (LH), and follicle-stimulating hormone (FSH). GRH helps or stimulates in the production of luteinizing hormone and follicle-stimulating hormone. Luteinizing hormone stimulates the synthesis and secretion of testosterone by the Leydig cells of the testes, and FSH helps luteinizing hormone stimulate the Leydig cells into producing testosterone. FSH also aids other cells of the testes in producing sperm. Another hormone, prolactin, which is produced by the pituitary, interacts with these hormones to decrease testosterone levels. Impotence may follow if there is underproduction of FSH, LH, gonadotropin-releasing hormone, or testosterone or if there is overproduction of prolactin.

June and Barbara: The vascular system is also a prime player in the sexual game. What is its function?

Dr. Lodewick: Ultimately what makes the penis become erect and firm is a good blood supply from the penile artery. The penis is composed of three anatomical cylinders. One contains the corpus spongiosum, which contains the urethra and permits the flow of urine and ejaculate. The other two cylinders, called the corpora cavernosa, occupy most of the space of the penis. During erection, these cylinders fill with blood from the penile artery to produce firmness and rigidity.

Smoking, alcohol, drugs, and hardening of the arteries may block this artery and prevent the penis from going up to allow for penetration. If the blood pressure gets too low (maybe from treatment of hypertension), it won't go up, either. Sometimes the veins can be a problem, too. If the veins in the penis don't close, the penis may go up but will then go down too quickly. The nervous system may also be involved here.

June and Barbara: What is the nervous system's involvement?

Dr. Lodewick: The nervous system is the initiator of the chain of events and is crucial for the climactic ending of a satisfactory sexual experience. It causes the vascular system to work correctly to engorge the penis. It's needed to experience good sensation and to allow the mind to carry on its activity. The nervous system can be impaired at any level and this could impair erection.

June and Barbara: Probably the only way to find the culprit in the impotence mystery is to have a medical evaluation. Just what does this entail?

Dr. Lodewick: A medical evaluation aimed at finding the answer to sexual dysfunction can range from minimal to complex—and the cost can range anywhere from $200 to more than $1000. However, it is important to find the cause because it will indicate the appropriate treatment or treatments and the possibility of a cure.

First, the history of the problem is reviewed with a physician. It is important for a diabetic man to bring up the problem himself, as many physicians aren't trained to initiate and discuss problems regarding sexuality. The history of impotence might give clues as to whether there is a psychological or medical component—or both. This involves reviewing the history of how diabetes has been managed, looking for medical problems such as hypertension that might be present, and ascertaining whether drugs (prescribed or illegal) or smoking is involved. This should be followed by a medical examination that might show evidence of the presence of nerve or vascular disease or hypertension.

At this point any psychological problems related to depression, anxiety, or medical problems that are apparent can be worked on. If a few visits to the doctor don't seem to resolve the problem, and both the man and his spouse agree, further investigation and tests are in order.

June and Barbara: What are some other significant tests that could give insights into sexual dysfunction?

Dr. Lodewick: One is the glycohemoglobin test; if it shows diabetes control is poor, this may explain why erection isn't taking place. Others include liver and kidney tests, cholesterol tests (HDL and LDL), and an electrocardiogram to gauge overall health. If he has liver, kidney, or heart disease, impotence may develop or result. If these are okay, then it may also be necessary to measure the male hormone testosterone, as well as prolactin, FSH, and LH. Remember, a man can feel fine and still have considerable underlying disease that is not apparent to him but that may be discernible to a physician after these tests.

Next, there is a significant test called measurement of penile erection. It's obviously important to find out at the onset if a man is capable of erection. A man may think that he isn't, yet he may actually still be. This is particularly true when there are psychological factors such as anxiety about performance, depression, and so on. This kind of test is a way of determining if the impotence is primarily psychological rather than physical.

A normal man has an average of four episodes of erection a night, each lasting 15 to 45 minutes. These are referred to medically as "nocturnal penile tumescence" and usually occur in conjunction with dreams. Incidentally, the nature of these dreams is not known, but they no doubt include some of one's own "creative erotic material." Finally, not only do the dreams cause erection, but it is normal for a man to wake up in the morning with an erection—the climax of a good night's sexual activity.

June and Barbara: Wouldn't a man be aware that all of these nocturnal goings-on are going on?

Dr. Lodewick: Not necessarily. Despite the richness and variety of his sexual activity in the arms of Morpheus, once he wakes up, he may not be aware that it happened. Since the mechanism for nocturnal penile erection is presumed to be identical to sexually stimulated erection, it's important to determine if he does have this activity. If he does, it points to a psychological cause for his sexual dysfunction, not a physical cause.

June and Barbara: How do you determine if these erections are indeed taking place?

Dr. Lodewick: There are several techniques. One way is relatively simple and involves placing a "snap gauge" around the penis at night. If the penis gets enlarged and rigid enough for intercourse, bands on the gauge will snap. The cost of this gauge generally runs $30 to $50. Some wise and thrifty patients substitute stamps for the snap gauge. Postage stamps or, for the truly thrifty, holiday seals, are wrapped around the penis at night and sealed together. If the stamps break at night, erection has occurred.

June and Barbara: On the chance that the general thrashing around of a sleepless or dream-filled night might cause the snap gauge to snap or the stamps to break, isn't there a more scientifically accurate test?

Dr. Lodewick: Yes, there is a more definitive and detailed (and more expensive) evaluation of erectile ability. This is done in a sleep laboratory over a two- to three-day period. Here the patient is observed while his penis is monitored for changes in circumference and firmness as measured by a mercury strain gauge transducer. This sleep laboratory investigation may cost from $800 to $1000.

A newer device that has become available over the past few years is the Rigiscan (from Dacomed Corporation, Minneapolis). It is a portable unit that can effectively do the same measurement of erectile ability on an ambulatory basis. A physician can arrange for a man to bring this ambulatory monitor home with him, and it gives him the advantage of monitoring his nocturnal penile tumescence activity in the privacy of his own home.

The information derived from the sleep laboratory or from a Rigiscan is frequently helpful not only for diagnostic purposes but also for educating the man as to the extent of his problem. This allows him and his spouse or partner to make a decision about whether to proceed with further testing or treatment.

June and Barbara: Let's say the nocturnal penile tumescence tests indicate that there is a physical basis for the impotence. What's the next step in the diagnostic detective work?

Dr. Lodewick: At this point, hormonal testing is in order. The tests would include blood testosterone levels and blood prolactin levels. If these prove to be abnormal, then tests for blood luteinizing hormone and follicle-stimulating hormone levels are needed. If testosterone and luteinizing hormone levels are low, the brain may not be producing them, which can occur in the presence of some generally benign tumors. This may require special X-rays and an eye exam, especially if the man has headaches and a high prolactin level.

June and Barbara: Since the vascular system is such a significant component of erection, what tests can be made to see if it's functioning properly?

Dr. Lodewick: There's a noninvasive test by means of Doppler ultrasonographic techniques. This compares the systolic blood pressure in the penile artery with that of the arm. If the ratio of these two blood pressures is less than 0.6, then it's a good chance that severe arterial disease is at fault. This could then be documented with a direct look at the arteries using a catheter and special dye. If significant vascular disease is present, surgery to open up the arteries may help.

If the penile blood pressure is good, but the penis doesn't remain erect long, this may indicate that the veins in the penis are draining the blood too quickly. This occurs in up to 15% or more of men with impotence. To look for this possibility, a study called cavernosometry and another called cavernosography may be needed. If this is present, inexpensive and simple ring bands (Confidence Rings by Performance Medical) are available that effectively restore the ability to maintain an erection.

June and Barbara: If none of these is at fault, that leaves us with nerve damage as the possible culprit.

Dr. Lodewick: That's right. The penis has to have good nerve sensation to work as it should. Impotence caused by nervous system involvement can be detected by an electromyogram or a pudendal nerve latency time test. If the nerves that transmit impulses necessary for erection (including the dorsal nerve to the penis and the bulbocavernous nerves) are working right, then erection will be possible.

June and Barbara: We strongly suspect that many diabetic men are hesitant to even discuss their impotence, or fears of impotence, with health professionals.

Dr. Lodewick: Your suspicions are correct. Most men don't discuss impotence for several reasons:

1. They don't realize that there are ways to help correct the problem, so their attitude is, "What's the use of even bringing up the subject?" In a survey of over 700 men conducted by the Opinion Research Corporation of Princeton, N.J., the majority of the men weren't aware of all the solutions currently available for impotence. An overwhelming number of them said they would seek treatment from a physician if they knew a solution were possible.

2. Many men are sexually modest and, although liking a good sexual relationship, think that their physicians will get the wrong idea about them. They're simply embarrassed to talk about it.

3. Many physicians don't initiate conversation about sexuality because they, themselves, may be too modest or because they're so busy working on acute medical problems that they don't have the time to discuss the possible emotional problems of sexual dysfunction.

June and Barbara: Some statistics from a seminar on impotence we attended in Detroit bear out all of your statements. When participants were asked, "What treatment options for impotence, if any, do you know of?" 69% said, "None." When asked, "If you found out your impotence was caused by a physical problem, would you seek treatment from a physician to correct the impotence problem?" 95% said, "Yes."

When asked, "Suppose you were impotent at this time; what would be your single biggest fear about seeking help for your impotence from a physician?" 45% responded, "The fear that there would be no solution." Another 25% said, "The fear that surgery would be required," while another 25% feared that it would be due to a physical cause. Finally, 20% were afraid of having the discussion with the doctor. (The reason this adds up to over 100% is that more than one answer was possible.)

Assuming that a man lacks this vital information, where—other than to his own physician—can he go for information, support, and for referrals to specialists and programs on impotence?

Dr. Lodewick: The following organizations are reliable sources for information and may be able to refer a diabetic man to a knowledgeable specialist.

Impotence Anonymous

There are 100 chapters nationwide. They provide self-help meetings on diagnosis and treatment. Contact Impotence Anonymous, 119 South Ruth St., Maryville, TN 37801.

National Kidney and Urologic Disease Information Clearing House

Provides a list of patient education material on impotence. For a free copy, write NKUDIC Impotence, Box NKUDIC, Bethesda, MD 20892.

Recovery of Male Potency

A self-help education program based in 27 hospitals. Contact Cindy Meredith, R.N., Grace Hospital, 18700 Meyers Road, Detroit, MI 48235, or call 1-800-835-7667 from anywhere in the United States (or 1-313-357-1216 from Michigan).

June and Barbara: As we said earlier, all diabetics, both men and women, have a tendency to blame diabetes for everything bad that happens to them. Could this be what happens with impotence—a man thinking that his impotence is diabetes-induced when it has another cause entirely?

Dr. Lodewick: Yes, there are many other reasons for impotence that have nothing to do with diabetes. Fortunately, many of these can be eliminated.

SMOKING

If you smoke—stop! In addition to all the other well-publicized medical reasons not to smoke, it causes constriction and hardening of the arteries. By impeding blood flow in the arteries to the penis, it may result in impotence. By giving up smoking, your breath will be cleaner, which will also make you more sexually appealing. I wish the information on smoking as a cause of impotence were more widely disseminated. It might help more than threats of lung cancer to make men give up the habit!

ALCOHOL AND ILLICIT DRUGS

The use of alcohol and illicit drugs such as marijuana and cocaine can have an adverse effect on sexual potency. (As Shakespeare said, "It increaseth the desire but decreaseth the performance.") When the libido is increased, it is frustrating to find out that no action follows—either because erection doesn't take place or because the woman won't respond to an intoxicated, sex-driven, unaffectionate, unromantic beast.

MEDICATIONS

Some legitimate medications can adversely affect erection (see listing in Appendix H). There are probably over 100 of them. Noteworthy and commonly used are blood pressure medications such as beta-blockers, Aldomet, and diuretics; antidepressants such as Elavil and Norpramine; ulcer medications such as Tagamet and Zantac; and medicines to prevent vomiting such as Reglan. Many of these and other medicines work by affecting the psychological, humoral (circulatory), and nervous pathways needed for erection. If you are on any of these medications, please discuss this possibility with your doctor; a change in medication to another equally effective one may help.

June and Barbara: We're always harping on the importance of good diabetes control as the solution to almost all problems a diabetic may encounter. Do you feel that impotence falls into that category? Can it often be reversed by maintaining normal blood sugars?

Dr. Lodewick: One of the first problems for a doctor to look for when a diabetic man develops impotence is poor control of his diabetes. I've seen many men with very poor diabetes control who have become transiently impotent. The difficulty here is that many times control is poor yet the man is not aware of it. The blood sugar can be as high as 250 mg/dl or more and yet give no major symptoms or clues that it is that high. This is why it's important to do self-testing of blood sugar faithfully. Under circumstances of poor control, the body is sapped of energy, the muscles lose strength, and eventually the man will suffer chronic fatigue and depression. Such men are in no mood for sex. Improved diabetes control will reverse this condition in many instances as long as the poor control has been short term. Thus, it's certainly possible in many cases that controlling the diabetes will alleviate the impotence.

June and Barbara: We've heard it said that sex is 90% above the neck. Consequently, we would expect that psychological factors are often totally or partially responsible for impotence in diabetic men. Could you fill us in on the psychological (psychogenic) aspects of diabetic impotence?

Dr. Lodewick: It's true that up there above the neck, the mind can do amazing things. There's a nerve pathway from the brain to the penis that responds to psychological stimulation and causes erection to take place. No physical stimulation is needed. Love is not needed. Just the sight or thought of a woman may send this pathway off to sexual stimulation. Unfortunately, psychological factors may also plague the mind so that this pathway can be blocked.

In men who have diabetes, psychological factors may well be implicated. The history of the impotence is important. If the onset of impotence was very abrupt, it suggests a psychogenic cause, whereas a gradual onset suggests a medical cause. If the problem is intermittent, occurring in some situations but not in others (or with some sexual partners but not with others), then a psychogenic cause is more probable. If the problem is constant, an underlying medical reason is more likely.

Other questions to help pinpoint whether there is a psychological versus a medical cause include whether or not erections occur at night or on awakening (95% of normal men wake up with an erection) and whether masturbation or pornography stimulates an erection. If erection occurs under these circumstances, a psychogenic cause is probable.

June and Barbara: What could be some of the underlying reasons for psychological causes of impotence?

Dr. Lodewick: Many of life's events can cause erectile difficulties. Since every man is different, some of these events can cause problems in one man but not in another. In general, an intact sense of masculinity is crucial, but what each man needs to feel masculine varies. There are men who feel that they have to be perfect physical specimens and 100% healthy or else they are "inadequate." These men (and there are untold numbers of them) think of themselves as never being suscep-tible to disease or injury. Even a minor injury such as a sprain after a ball game may jar their sense of masculinity and, at least temporarily, cause problems with erection. If a more serious illness such as diabetes occurs, they may have a terrible time coming to grips with it and more prolonged sexual difficulties may follow.

In a similar fashion, since many men look upon their careers as the core of their lives, any adverse, unlucky, or stressful situation affecting their careers may make men look upon themselves as failures. Not getting a raise or promotion or being viewed unfavorably by colleagues or superiors may also have this negative effect on their sex lives. Outside the career, a financial setback can have a major effect on a man's self-esteem since wealth is looked upon (at least in the United States) as a measure of one's success.

The most obvious cause of sexual dysfunction is marital woes. An emotional fight, the wife's prompting of the husband to be a better lover (making him wonder who his wife is comparing him to), or a husband's affair causing guilt and anxiety and depression are all causes for concern and remedy.

I've seen a number of widowers who had sexual problems that didn't become apparent until after their wives died and they met new women. Some of these men had been very loving and devoted husbands and either felt guilty over finding a new woman or, because of anxiety, weren't sure they could perform adequately to satisfy their new partners. Divorce stemming from a wife's unfaithfulness could result in similar sexual anxiety that could cause sexual difficulties.

As you might imagine, retirement could well be associated with a decline in a man's self-esteem and masculinity. This is especially true if, as in so many men's lives, their careers have been successful and a major source of prestige. Also, mental illness or states such as depression may decrease libido and therefore decrease sexual interaction. Obviously, there are many other possible psychological factors that could contribute to impotence that a diabetic man experiencing them might know better than I.

June and Barbara: Does psychological counseling really work if the impotence is psychological in nature?

Dr. Lodewick: If the history and physical exam suggest a nonmedical reason for impotence, psychological therapy may be a first-line approach. This is especially true if the nighttime penile tumescence shows the degree, frequency, and duration of erections to be first rate. Dr. Charles Fisher, M.D., Director of the Sleep Laboratory at the Mount Sinai School of Medicine, notes that in his experience, almost all patients with psychological impotence have good nocturnal penile erections. So, if a man has good erections at night, he should also be able to have them with conscious sexual contact. It is estimated that 75% of men with psychological impotence will respond to sexual counseling with increased performance.

June and Barbara: When there are medical problems causing the impotence and it becomes apparent that these problems can't be reversed with improved diabetes control, what should a man do?

Dr. Lodewick: For impotence that cannot be reversed, there are many possible solutions, up to and including a penile implant. But before resorting to surgery, there are several external devices a man should first consider. Personally, I would recommend trying these, as they give the couple the chance to evaluate the resumption of sexual intercourse, to see how it feels again after living without it for such a long time.

June and Barbara: What are these external devices, how do they work, and how effective are they?

Dr. Lodewick: There are basically two different types of external devices; one is referred to as a vacuum entrapment (or vacuum constricting device) and the other is a vacuum nonentrapment device.

Vacuum constriction is a method of treating partial or complete impotence. It has been known to the scientific community for many years. The basic concept of this therapy is that a vacuum is used to assist filling when there is failure to fill, while a constriction device assists when there is a failure to hold. The constriction helps to hold the erection by constricting the veins. These two approaches combined have been able to offer success to more than 80% of the patients who have used them. There are currently several of these types of devices available. One, called the ErecAid, is made by Osbon (Osbon Medical Systems, P.O. Drawer 1478, Augusta, GA 30903; 1-800-438-8592). Another, the Response System, is manufactured by Smith-Collins Pharmaceutical (889 South Matlack Street, West Chester, PA; 1-800-444-5748). A third unit, called the Post-T-Vac, is manufactured by Post-T-Vac, Inc. (P.O. Box 1436DF, Dodge City, KS 67801; 1-800-627-7434), and a fourth, the Performance Plus Method (EID or Erection Inducer Device and Confidence Rings), is by Performance Medical (100 Dobbs Lane, Suite 205, Cherry Hill, NJ 08034; 1-609-354-8154 for information; 1-800-877-7420 for ordering).

A typical vacuum constrictor system consists of a cylinder that is placed over the penis; a vacuum pump, which is used to draw air out of the cylinder; and a constriction band, which is used to hold blood within the penis. The constricting band is placed over the cylinder, which is then placed over the flaccid (resting) penis. Upon operation of the pump, air is drawn out of the cylinder, causing blood to flow into the penis.

When sufficient blood has entered the penis, it will become engorged and rigid. At this point, the constriction band is guided manually from the cylinder to the base of the erect penis, the vacuum is released, and the cylinder is removed. A man can maintain this erection-like state, adequate for vaginal penetration, as long as a properly fitted constriction band is in place.

Vacuum constrictors became commercially available in 1974 when Osbon released the first system into the marketplace. Since that time, it is estimated that in excess of 50,000 such systems have been used. In the wake of this initial offering, several firms have entered the marketplace offering devices similar to Osbon's. Of these competitors, only one firm has offered more than one type of system, and that same firm offers several unique devices that appear to improve safety, performance, and ease of use. Within the last year, Smith-Collins Pharmaceutical, of West Chester, Pennsylvania, has increased its offering to a total of four systems by adding three new systems to its original patented system.

Beginning in 1987, Smith-Collins offered a vacuum device that was substantially easier to use than the systems existing at that time. Based on the patented and efficient diaphragm pump mechanism, this system can be operated with only one hand, in contrast to the rather unwieldy two-handed devices of other systems. This system was greeted with much success and has led to the development of a rechargeable battery system that is even easier to use. This new system, called the Touch System, is a streamlined, one-handed device that offers the greatest ease of any on the market. Quiet and safe (the vacuum pressure is limited to 250 mmHg as suggested by some studies), this device is reasonably priced; in fact, it is just a few dollars more than some of the older generation pumps—generally around $300 to $425.

In contrast to some of the other systems, the Smith-Collins systems also have numerous safety advantages. All of them are based on a unique soft, wide constriction ring that is specifically fitted to the individual. Other manufacturers of vacuum constrictor systems provide very narrow rings or rubber bands or both. While the risk of injury with any of the devices is very low, it appears that the Smith-Collins rings offer greater comfort to the user as well as a greater likelihood of maintaining an erection. This is because of the wide cross-sectional area that the rings cover, thereby allowing constriction to take place across a greater area of the penis, thus improving the likelihood of success.

A second unique feature of these systems is the built-in vacuum release valve. The safety valve feature also allows for the vacuum to be released easily after the constriction band is applied. Alternately, the vacuum release valve may be used for the suggested regimen of pumping and releasing the vacuum to enhance the function of the vascular system. Several informal studies have indicated that such a regimen may offer a means of rebuilding the vascular system of certain patients. To the extent that a given patient can benefit from this exercise, the Response System products make it both simple and safe.

In addition to three types of pumps for vacuum constriction, Smith-Collins also offers a device for men who can obtain an erection but are unable to maintain it. This system, called the Restore System, is based on the same rings and components as the vacuum systems. By using a collar to enable the patient to apply a constrictor ring, the Restore System uses the constriction concept alone without the use of a vacuum device.

Just released in 1990 is yet another very easy-to-use vacuum device: the EID (Erection Inducer Device) made by Performance Medical (1-800-877-7920). This costs about $350 and includes the uniquely formulated Confidence Rings that allow for normal ejaculation. The Confidence Rings can also be purchased separately ($50 for a set of two rings) and used to maintain erections in men who have rapid leaking of the veins.

The effectiveness of any of these devices can be expected to improve with practice. Some studies have indicated significant improvement after one or two weeks of continued use. Similarly, the involvement of the partner with the use of these systems has also been shown to improve the success rate.

June and Barbara: Have any of your own patients achieved success with these vacuum constriction systems?

Dr. Lodewick: Many have. This report of one patient who used the Post-T-Vac is a typical experience.

> Having been married for 23 years and single for another 6½ years, I found upon remarriage that I was almost entirely unable to perform sexually. After several months of hormonal and medicinal treatments that did not work, it was suggested

that I try vacuum therapy. I was skeptical about this type of treatment with which I was totally unfamiliar.

The results we attained with Post-T-Vac were amazing to both me and my wife. I went from almost total inability to superability. Using this vacuum pump has improved my natural abilities and the way I was feeling about myself.

I am so thankful that we learned about this therapy, and I would recommend it for many sufferers of impotence. It may not solve everyone's problem of impotence, but I am sure that many would be delighted with the results.

There are some potential problems with these entrapment devices. One, the bands entrap blood and could therefore disturb blood flow, especially after orgasm. This could be a problem. In addition, they may prevent ejaculation. And for men with bleeding troubles, they could cause bleeding. For all of these reasons, they should not be used unwisely nor for more than about 15 minutes at a time, and not without the direction of a knowledgeable doctor.

To get more detailed information about these devices, you can ask your doctor or, if he or she doesn't have a complete file, write to the Impotence Institute of America (IIA, Inc.), a nonprofit organization dedicated to allow both lay persons and health-care professionals access to information. Their address is IIA, Inc., 119 South Ruth St., Maryville, TN, 37801-5746.

June and Barbara: Moving along to the second type of external device, what is a vacuum nonentrapment device and how is it used?

Dr. Lodewick: A nonentrapment device is one that does not entrap blood in the penis with a constrictor ring. An example of this would be the condom device called the Synergist Erection Device manufactured by Synergist Limited (6910 Fannin, Suite 100, Houston, TX 77030; 1-800-422-9005). This is by far the easiest and least complicated of all the devices. It is a custom-fitted penile sheath made of soft, transparent silicone rubber. It appears very much like a condom so it is aesthetically acceptable. When placed over the penis, it creates a vacuum by applying suction. The sheath has a thin, pliable collar that seals the vacuum at the base of the penis. Since this collar does not constrict the penis, the device can be worn for 15 to 30 minutes or more—plenty of time to ensure the partner's sexual satisfaction. And because the condom covers the penis, there is no chance of sexually transmitted disease.

In one medical report of 12 diabetic men with impotence of three years' duration, all were able to have erections after using the Synergist device. There were no side effects when the men used it an average of two times a month over a three-month period. Most of the men were satisfied with the device. Their only complaint was a diminished sensation for themselves. It was with the use of this device that one of my patients concluded, "The resumption of our sexual relationship made the difference of night and day."

I would certainly recommend this as a possible solution before considering the major step of a penile implant (surgery).

June and Barbara: Are there any other possible solutions to try before entering into surgery?

Dr. Lodewick: There are two: Yohimbine and penile injections.

A MEDICINE THAT WORKS—YOHIMBINE

Yohimbine is a prescription medicine that stimulates the mood and—in a small percentage of patients reported to have a medical reason for impotence—can even stimulate the penis as well by stimulating blood flow. It is taken three times per day, usually over a six-month period. It may have some minor side effects, so you need to discuss these with your doctor.

PENILE INJECTIONS

In the last few years, an injection directly into the base of the penis of some medicines that increase blood flow into that area have been used. These medications include papaverine and phentolamine. They are injected with an insulin syringe into the corpora cavernosa, which are the cylinders adjacent to the urethra in the penis. These fill with blood in an erection. Although some patients have reported satisfaction with this technique, I'm not sure of the possible long-range complications, and most men would prefer stimulation of their penis by a far more normal technique—a female companion. As with all of these treatments for impotence, injections should be thoroughly discussed with your doctor so that you are aware of any potential side effects or interactions with other drugs you may be taking.

June and Barbara: Now we come to the impotence court of last resort—penile implants. When would you suggest that a man consider this measure?

Dr. Lodewick: A man might consider a penile implant after it has been definitely determined that his sexual dysfunction is not reversible by any simpler means. Even then, before electing surgery, he should explore marital, sex, and/or psychiatric therapy. I want to emphasize that a successful penile implant may not by itself improve the relationship.

The man and his wife should be aware of the advantages and disadvantages and possible complications and risks of each type of implant. Ideally, the man should have a strong libido and a desiring sexual partner and be reasonably healthy. It may be helpful for him to discuss this prospective surgery with a patient who has already had the same kind of surgical implant.

Penile implants have been on the scene since the 1970s. More than 50,000 diabetic men have received them. If successful, this solution to impotence is probably the best, since the man is always ready for lovemaking, never having to worry about having his external device along with him when the time is right. In fact, even when the man is not in the mood—for example, right after a successful sexual encounter—he may satisfy his partner even more with continued erectile functioning. As one of my patients put it, "It's better now than even before I became impotent." His wife echoed his sentiment.

June and Barbara: You mention that a candidate for a penile implant should discuss the prospective surgery with someone who has had the same kind of implant. Is there more than one kind?

Dr. Lodewick: There are two types of penile prostheses: inflatable and semirigid.

INFLATABLE PENILE IMPLANTS

The inflatable prostheses attempt to provide the patient with the most natural appearing and functional phallus, in both the erect and flaccid state. The body's natural erectile process is a hydraulic phenomenon; the inflatable prosthesis works on this same basis. In addition, the prosthesis does nothing to interfere with the natural mechanisms involved in intercourse, orgasm, or ejaculation.

If there is no nerve damage due to diabetes, men should have reasonably normal sensations during intercourse. In addition, if ejaculation and orgasm were achievable prior to the implant, the same will be true afterward. Even fathering a child is possible in contrast to what happens with some of the external devices, which may block the ejaculate.

Some of the inflatable penile prostheses consist of inflatable penile cylinders, a pump for inflation and deflation, and a fluid reservoir. The cylinders are inserted into the corpora cavernosa. The pump is placed in the scrotum, and when it is squeezed, it sends the reservoir fluid to the penile cylinders, causing erection. The reservoir is inserted into the abdomen. One such inflatable penile implant, called the AMS 700 CX, is produced by American Medical Systems (1-800-328-3881).

The more recently devised prostheses are smaller and self-contained so they are easier to insert because only one rod lies in the length of the penis and a scrotal pump is not needed. One such device, also made by American Medical Systems, is called the Hydroflex; another made by Surgitek (1-800-328-3863) is called the Flexi-flate. The cost of all these implants—including surgery—generally runs $3000 to $5000.

SEMIRIGID PENILE IMPLANTS

There are several types of semirigid implants that can be inserted into the corpora cavernosa. It is a very simple surgical procedure to insert these into the penis, and therefore they can be done on an outpatient basis for about $1000. These implants come in varying lengths and diameters so that they can be custom fitted. They are made of silicone material, and the latest models are flexible and bendable to help with concealment when not being used, but they are still difficult to conceal totally—an obvious disadvantage. There is the Small-Carrion made by Mentor, the Flexi-rod made by Surgitek, the ESKA Jonas Silicone Siver made by C. R. Bard, and the AMS 600 made by American Medical Systems. The urologist who performs the surgery should be able to give the benefits of each type.

June and Barbara: Are there some potential problems with surgical implants?

Dr. Lodewick: The disadvantage of this method of treatment is that there is surgery involved. With any surgery, complications are possible, even infections in up to 2% of patients. If infection occurs, the prosthesis may need to be removed and reimplantation would be more difficult. Loss of penile tissue may also occur. Also, about 3% of men report pain with intercourse.

Therefore, before a man considers this surgery, he should make sure he has good diabetes control and is in as good physical condition as possible. He should be aware that the devices may need repair or replacement after five to seven years. According to one diabetes article, satisfactory results from penile implants are about 80 to 90%.

Incidentally, the Grace Hospital in Detroit, Michigan reports in its brochure *Solving the Problem of Impotence* that men as young as 15 and as old as 94 have received penile implants. The statistical breakdown on implants by age is as follows:

Under age 20:	0.17%
20–29:	3.3%
30–39:	7.3%
40–49:	13.9%
50–59:	31.3%
60–69:	33.4%
70–79:	10.2%
80–89:	0.48%

June and Barbara: Many men profess to want to cure their impotence for the benefit of the women in their lives, but a Dear Abby survey once reported that most women prefer cuddling to actual sex. If men aren't truly going through the impotence treatment for themselves, wouldn't it be a good idea for the couple to have counseling with a sex therapist to ascertain what each partner really wants? That way they could see if alternative ways of achieving satisfaction are possible, especially in cases where the only treatment possible for the man is surgery.

Dr. Lodewick: There is no simple answer to this question. The survey may even be biased. It may have been answered mainly by women whose relationships with the men in their lives have been less than loving ones, so that the women have the attitude that "all men are interested in is sex." If the men in their lives are, in fact, not providing these women with all the other satisfactions of a loving male–female relationship, including hugging, touching, cuddling, and tenderness in words and action, then it certainly would be advisable to have sexual counseling and probably marriage counseling prior to considering penile surgery.

In my survey of patients, I've found that a woman may like the sexual act more than the man or it may be the other way around. In a truly loving relationship where physical impotence is present, a man may feel that he wants to give his partner full sexual satisfaction. Under such circumstances, it may be advisable before considering surgery for a sex counselor to help ascertain how necessary it is to complete the full sexual act through intercourse with a total erection. Many women who are in love with their men may be content with just cuddling. Other women, if they want orgasmic pleasure, can actually derive it from their men in many ways without a fully erect penis. If these women and their men don't know how to give each other such sexual pleasure without full intercourse, a sex counselor may help them learn how. If, however, the woman desires the full sexual act, then impotence treatment should be considered.

In some cases, men feel that their wives are just being kind in denying their needs because they don't want to deflate their male egos. These men are very gratified in being able to resume intercourse with an erect penis. So surgery may be their only solution.

I would conclude by saying that the most important thing in this circumstance is to find out what each partner truly desires. After appropriate discussion and possibly sex counseling, then a good decision can be made about surgery or an alternative treatment for the man.

June and Barbara: Although the problem of impotence looms as the major concern of a diabetic man, there are other aspects of his sexuality that need consideration. For example, one of the letters we received in response to our request for questions from diabetic men dealt with the decision to have a vasectomy.

> Since my wife and I are 38 years old and feel that our family is complete, I have been considering a vasectomy as a means of permanent birth control. I had felt a vasectomy was probably the best choice for us until I read *Is Vasectomy Safe?* by H. J. Roberts, M.D. He cites case histories of postvasectomy thrombophlebitis, reactive hypoglycemia, atherosclerosis, and other vascular diseases. He also suggests that sperm antigens may react with different organs and interfere with the natural immune response. Roberts believes that diabetes mellitus puts one in the "high risk" group for postvasectomy complications.
>
> I asked the public library to check the literature for any research about vasectomy and its relation to diabetes. Their computer search of 1983 to the present failed to find any journal articles on this topic.
>
> I realize that it's possible I can read just enough to scare myself, but I am now more cautious about a vasectomy realizing that diabetes is an autoimmune disease and that a vasectomy would create another kind of autoimmune response (that is, the formation of sperm antibodies to deal with the sperm that are continually produced).
>
> I have posed this question to two doctors and received two answers: "Vasectomies are safe for diabetics" and "Vasectomies are not safe for diabetics."
>
> I would very much appreciate your opinion about the safety of vasectomy surgery and would be very grateful for any thoughts you could share on this matter.

Dr. Lodewick: It is a wise decision for a diabetic man to be as informed as possible concerning a vasectomy.

Vasectomy is a very common procedure. It has been used since the 1800s as a form of birth control and for other not so valid reasons. In the United States it is estimated that 250,000 to 500,000 men have this procedure done each year. Over 12,000,000 men have already had it done. Although complications can occur as with any surgery, according to *Current Therapy in Endocrinology and Metabolism*, over a dozen long-term studies of a large number of men have failed to detect any long-term consequences.

The procedure itself is simple and can be performed on an outpatient basis using local anesthesia. A small cut is made through the vas deferens, which is a tiny tube leading from the epididymus (an elongated organ at the bottom of a testis) to the ejaculatory ducts in the penis. The passage of motile sperm from the testes and epididymus is thus prevented from getting to the ejaculatory ducts. Within 90 days, over 90% of men no longer produce sperm. In the hands of a good urologist, surgeon, or well-experienced family physician, the complication rates are extremely low. In one survey of over 5,000 patients, only 13 major complications occurred. Minor complications include infection and bleeding at the surgical site.

There have been some fears of long-term complications. Accelerated arteriosclerosis was reported in monkeys after vasectomy. On further review of these monkeys, it was found that they were on a fat-filled diet. The latest *Scientific American* medical reports state that at this point, accelerated arteriosclerosis has not been proven. This article also reports that in another study there was no increased incidence in heart disease in men 10 years after vasectomy.

Reactive hypoglycemia is of no concern to a diabetic because this is a condition in nondiabetics that can be prevented by a good diet. It is not seen in insulin-dependent diabetics because it is caused by too much insulin being released from the pancreas. Thrombophlebitis is very unlikely because with good surgical technique, it happens very rarely. The last problem mentioned in the letter concerning sperm antigens is only hypothetical. The idea here is when the vas deferens is cut, the sperm may be exposed to the main bloodstream and be thought of as foreign to the body and affect the immune system. So far, no disturbances to the immune system have been documented to cause any complications.

Among my patients who have undergone the procedure, I have seen no significant complications that I could attribute to it. There is the possibility that some unforeseen complication may occur many years after vasectomy, but if that does occur, it would not be predicted on the basis of our present state of knowledge about this relatively simple operation.

June and Barbara: We received one very poignant letter from a woman about her diabetic sweetheart of 3 years. He is a Type I diabetic, 45 years old, and has been blind from retinopathy for 18 years. Many of her questions dealt with topics in your discussion of impotence, but she had another: "He gets yeast on his beast! He uses Micatin. Is this the best product? I think that sometimes we pass it back and forth without realizing it. Condoms aren't too good, especially for the reason I mentioned above. (He gets erections, but it takes a long time and a lot of stimulation for him to have an orgasm by any means, more so to have intercourse.)"

We realize that diabetic women often have problems with yeast infections, but we didn't realize that diabetic men are susceptible as well.

Dr. Lodewick: Although men don't have yeast infections as frequently as women, they *do* have them. They are usually related to poor diabetes control and/or complications. Generally when diabetes is well controlled and uncomplicated, a yeast infection will disappear with the use of Micatin (or Mycolog or Monostat creams) and will not return.

June and Barbara: This correspondent also mentioned that "his fingers aren't too sensitive." There may be some neuropathy, but we think his fingers have calluses from being stuck at least four times a day for his blood sugar tests. Any suggestions for that problem?

Dr. Lodewick: The loss of sensation is most likely from neuropathy and not from calluses. The important thing for neuropathy is to work on good diabetes control, and to do that you must do frequent blood sugar testing.

June and Barbara: And now for a final major sexual concern for the diabetic man: can diabetes cause sterility?

Dr. Lodewick: Diabetes doesn't generally cause sterility directly. A healthy diabetic man can be virile, have plenty of male hormone (testosterone), and have libido and potency. However, when diabetes affects the nervous and/or vascular system to the extent that a man is impotent, then ejaculation may not be as good as it should and the man becomes infertile. Sometimes, even when there are no problems with potency, an ejaculation may go back into the bladder rather than forward into the vagina (retrograde ejaculation). In the case of either impotence or retrograde ejaculation, it is still possible to obtain sperm and inseminate the spouse artificially.

When the wife is having a problem becoming pregnant, she may need evaluation, too. Sometimes both the wife and the husband are contributing to the dilemma, as illustrated by the case of Jan and Joe who begat Sarah.

Jan had a problem with an irregular menstrual cycle because her ovaries were not working right. The problem of her diabetic husband Joe was that his sperm went back into his bladder instead of out his penis. While Jan's menstrual irregularity was treated so that her eggs would be produced on time, Joe's sperm was isolated right after it went into his bladder by having him urinate and saving the sperm in a saline solution. Jan was then inseminated with this solution, and one of these sperm met with her egg. Beautiful little Sarah was born as a result of this union. Sarah is now 10 years old.

By the way, Joe has had diabetes over 40 years now and is still going strong—sexually and in other areas of his life— without any major complications.

POSTSCRIPT

Don't Myth Out on Sex!

The *Kinsey Institute New Report on Sex* reveals that of 2000 American adults who were asked 18 true–false and multiple choice questions on sex, only 45% could answer 10 or more correctly. The Kinsey folks concluded that there is a lot of sexual misinformation floating around out there. One of the widely accepted myths is that impotence usually cannot be treated successfully. Wrong! According to the study, it's frequently a physical problem that can be fixed. This confirms what you've just read in this chapter—and now you know all the different ways it can be fixed.

Another important bit of information from the Kinsey report is that sexual activity both before and after orgasm burns up 6.4 calories per minute. This might prove to be a popular inclusion in weight-reduction programs for Type II men. And Type I men should take note that 10 minutes of foreplay or afterplay uses up one fruit exchange (60 calories, 15 grams carbohydrate). A final glad tiding is that the belief that sex usually ends soon after age 60 is totally false.

The report also points out that it is perfectly normal to sometimes cry after orgasm. This puts us in mind of a wry quote attributed to the actress Glenda Jackson: "The important thing in acting is to be able to laugh and cry. If I have to cry, I think of my sex life. If I have to laugh, I think of my sex life." We trust that after heeding the advice in this chapter and dispelling all your negative myths, in the future when you think of your sex life, you will neither laugh nor cry, but will just smile. . . knowingly!

The
TRAVELING MAN
· · · ·
Shape Up and Ship Out

Aside from emergency family obligations, there are two basic reasons to travel: for love or for money. If you're in the first category and travel because you love it, travel is one of the great, mind-expanding joys of your life. You may find that traveling sparks your creativity. In her book *Uncommon Genius: How Great Ideas Are Born*, Denise Shekerjian points out the importance of play—of being able to relax and have a good time—and the importance of travel, if for no other reason than the off chance of being inspired by new surroundings. (You may even find that your heightened creativity gives you innovative ideas on how to manage your diabetes.) Travel also increases your spontaneity quotient, giving you an ability to be light on your literal and figurative feet and make quick decisions. A diabetic stock trader we know likes spontaneous weekend get-aways. He goes to the airport, looks over the available flights and takes the first one that's going to a destination no more than two hours away. When he was first diagnosed diabetic, he was mourning over the fact that such weekend flights of fancy would be over because of his diabetes. When we asked why his diabetes would possibly stop him, he thought a couple of minutes and couldn't come up with any reason, so he's still leaping onto planes just as before.

The play and creative aspects of travel along with getting away from your daily grind of problems also serve to reduce stress—and as Dr. Lodewick repeatedly points out, stress is one of the greatest enemies of diabetes control.

The other kind of travel—traveling for money, better known as business travel—can be the antithesis of traveling for the love of it. Such obligatory travel can even be a grueling, loathsome grind. But there's often no way out. You may have to do it. In many lines of work, frequent travel is a requirement of the job, so that a man who refuses to travel could be stopped in his advancement track or even dismissed. The trick is to turn your business trip into somewhat of a pleasure by giving yourself small rewards along the way. Read up on the places you're visiting (it will impress your business associates when you know something about their community) and take a little time out to look around and see the sights when you get there. If it can be arranged, try to add a mini-vacation onto the end of a trip— for example, a weekend on nearby ski slopes after a business trip to Salt Lake City or a few rounds of golf or games of tennis after a conference in Phoenix. It's even better if you can arrange to have a wife or girlfriend, family member, or friend meet you or go with you. Having an amiable travel companion doubles the fun. But don't think of a travel companion as a diabetes necessity. As an independent, well-controlled diabetic you can take care of yourself when you travel as well as you can at home. You don't need someone hovering over you to remind you to eat, exercise, or take your medication.

Surprisingly enough, just as travel can make you a better-controlled diabetic, being a well-controlled diabetic can make you a better traveler. Travel requires fitness, what with all the running to catch planes and walking up stairs and hoisting luggage. Dr. Mary E. Wilson, chief of infectious diseases at Mount Auburn Hospital in Cambridge, Massachusetts, has this to say about travel:

> For people with a sedentary lifestyle, much of travel can be very strenuous. Walking even on level surfaces above sea level can put increased stress on the cardiovascular system. The days are long,

there is a change in the time zone, and moving from place to place creates its own stress.... If there are underlying cardiac and vascular problems, travelers feel fatigue. There may not be an increased likelihood of illness, but being tired hampers enjoyment.

Many people who are well in the sense that they don't have a chronic disease like diabetes are not very fit because of their sedentary lifestyles and their hauling around of several extra pounds. If you keep your diabetes in control with an exercise program (including aerobics) and a healthy diet, you will be fit and in shape to handle whatever travel has in store for you. As a well-controlled diabetic, you are also less likely to while away the hours aloft or waiting for flights with cocktails that can dull your mind and senses for business or pleasure.

Inveterate traveler Robert Louis Stevenson once said, "I travel not to go anywhere, but to go. I travel for travel's sake. The great affair is to move."

Don't let diabetes stop you. Move!

—*June and Barbara*

WHAT YOU'LL FIND HERE

SUPPLIES

AIRPORT SECURITY

INSULIN ADJUSTMENT AND TIME ZONE CHANGES

JET LAG

TRAVELING ALONE

EXERCISE

DINING OUT

AUTOMOBILE TRAVEL

BEACH VACATIONS

TRAVEL TIPS

June and Barbara: When June gets ready for a trip—even for a weekend—she starts packing her diabetes supplies at least a week ahead of time. She knows from experience that if she waits until the last minute, she is likely not to have something on hand that she needs to take. In the excitement of getting ready to go she may even forget something vital (just like the honeymooners our travel agent told us about who winged off to Tahiti without their birth control pills). She carries double diabetes supplies with her, keeping one set in her purse and one in the hand luggage she carries onto the plane. It's not a good idea to keep your diabetes supplies in the luggage you check because it may not arrive with you and because the cargo area of the plane may be either too cold or too hot.

Dr. Lodewick, we would like to know what personal travel methods you use to ensure that your diabetes will have a smooth trip.

Dr. Lodewick: One of the phrases I often remember from my Latin course prerequisite for medical school is *semper paratus*—always prepared. That's the motto of the U.S. Coast Guard and I make it mine when I travel. Knowledge and preparedness are crucial in ensuring an outstanding trip for an otherwise healthy diabetic man.

As far as diabetes supplies are concerned, it is most important to have enough. Bring extras of everything in case some are stolen, broken, or lost. Even one learned diabetic doctor with whom you are familiar has in the past suffered the inconvenience and embarrassment of getting caught short and has vowed never to let it happen again.

To carry my supplies I always try to wear clothing that allows me to keep them with me at all times. Fortunately, diabetes care supplies have become increasingly smaller and more convenient to carry. I like comfortable, loose-fitting clothing with plenty of pockets to put things in. Actually, army fatigues are perfect for travel, unless you're on a very important business trip and expect to be negotiating with someone other than Fidel Castro.

For casual occasions I usually wear shirts with two pockets that button to carry my NovoPen (a compact pen-sized insulin delivery device made by Novo-Nordisk) and blood-testing supplies. There are also some neat jackets and raincoats that provide plenty of storage space for more formal affairs. When I have on a tuxedo, I wear a shoulder holster to carry my needed supplies in an inconspicuous fashion.

June and Barbara: Speaking of supplies, could you give us a run-down on what the traveling man would be likely to take with him?

Dr. Lodewick: He needs all his diabetes supplies: insulin and syringes or oral diabetes medications, glucose tablets in case of low blood sugar (I prefer Dextrosols, those glucose tablets first recommended by my fellow diabetic doctor–writer, Richard K. Bernstein), and all the blood-testing paraphernalia to keep track of your blood sugar levels. It's better to know for sure what your blood sugar is than to guess at it; this avoids the embarrassment or reactions or the long-range problems of high blood sugar.

I've been fooled more than once upon finding my blood sugars surprisingly high when traveling despite the fact that I was eating less. It's been my experience that long rides in planes, trains, or cars will frequently cause my blood sugar to go high. Whether it's the excitement or stress of embarking on a trip or just the sitting around that is a consequence of traveling in a vehicle, the phenomenon is somewhat of a mystery. In cases such as these, I frequently cut my carbohydrate food intake substantially to avoid prolonged hyperglycemia.

A good idea for blood sugar testing—especially if you travel abroad and there is a question about the functioning of your meter—is always to take some visual test strips. You can resort to these if your meter isn't working, if you have some doubts about its accuracy, or if you break or lose it. (Incidentally, to keep a battery-operated meter working, bring along an extra battery.)

Also, especially for Type I men, you should bring along urine ketone test strips in case you get sick and your blood sugar goes unexpectedly high. If this test shows that ketones are high, with blood sugars above 240 mg/dl, extra Regular insulin may be needed. This is like the extra insulin you take when you're ill and showing ketones in your urine. Make sure before you leave that you learn how much and when to take extra Regular insulin in case of illness. Discuss this with your doctor.

Other possible general medical supplies to include are dramamine (which can make you very sleepy), bonine, or scopolamine patches for sea sickness or air sickness, as well as medicines to guard against and counteract illnesses resulting from drinking water in other countries, such as diarrhea, nausea, and abdominal cramping. (I recommend diphenoxylate, Lomotil, loperamide, or Imodium for diarrhea; Pepto-Bismol for nausea and cramping; and trimethobenzamide, Tigan, or compazine for vomiting.) Naturally, you shouldn't forget any other medicines that you may take on a regular basis. Check all these out with your doctor before you leave and also ask him or her about the possible need to bring along antibiotics in case of illness.

June and Barbara: On the subject of taking along your diabetes testing equipment and supplies, many diabetic travelers worry about damaging their blood sugar testing meters and strips going through airport security. To give you some guidelines on this, we asked Linda Naney, SugarFree Centers' Director of Outreach Services, to investigate. These are her findings.

Boehringer-Mannheim (makers of the Accu-Chek and Tracer) report that there is a possibility that the X-ray in an airport could zap out the calibration code. You might see three dashes (– – –) when you're ready to do a test, in which case you would have to recalibrate. In fact, it would be a good idea to recalibrate anyway after you've taken the meter through an X-ray. There is no problem with the strips going through the X-ray.

Home Diagnostics (makers of the Diascan and the Ultra) say that going through security does not hurt either the meter or the strips.

Ames (makers of Glucometer II and III) state that their meters and strips are not harmed by X-rays. There is, however, a possibility that X-rays could give the models with a memory a case of amnesia. Consequently, they suggest handing your memory meter to the attendant and not putting it through security check if you depend on your memory feature for your records. The meter, itself, will *not* be harmed. They also recommend checking calibration after a blast from the X-ray.

Lifescan (makers of Glucosan and One Touch) say neither their meters nor their strips have any problem going through airport security X-ray.

Medisense (makers of ExacTech and Companion) report that airport security will not affect either their meters or strips, but they say that you shouldn't put them in with your checked luggage because the cargo area may be too cold for them.

Elco (makers of Direct 30/30) say that it doesn't harm their meter or sensor to go through airport security.

June often has her Medi-Jector insulin jet injector in her hand luggage when she goes through airport security. Only once did they pick it up on the X-ray and make her open her bag and show it to them. They accepted her explanation without a quibble. Although it's nice to know that you don't have problems taking a jet injector along in your travels, we don't find it all that reassuring that airport security personnel routinely allow a metallic, torpedo-shaped device to slip through security without batting an eye. If this can get on board so easily, who knows what lethal weapons may get on board in hand luggage!

Even though she may have a jet injector in her hand luggage, June usually finds it easier to take her insulin with a needle when aloft. But if you do this, you must remember not to inject air into the insulin vial. If you do, the difference in air pressure in the cabin will cause the needle to "fight you" and make it hard to measure your correct dose.

Then the question arises as to where you should take your shot in a plane. A recently diagnosed New York stock trader of our acquaintance told us about his first experience of taking an insulin shot in public. It happened in a packed airplane. He was sandwiched in between two large men and didn't want to annoy them and the flight attendants by trying to get out of his seat and down the aisle to the lavatory before the food trays arrived. So he just turned to the two fellows and said, "You don't mind if I take a shot of insulin here, do you? I'd rather not have to disturb you by going back to the restroom." He was very relaxed and loose about it, and as a result, so were they. They just mumbled something like, "Go right ahead. Doesn't bother me" and returned to their reading. Now he just shoots sitting in his seat in airplanes all the time.

On the subject of insulin, Type I men often ask how they should adjust their insulin when they fly into different time zones. Some of the answers we've heard—and have sometimes given—are so complex and convoluted that you'd almost rather stay home or resort to traveling only north and south so you'd never change time zones and wouldn't have to adjust it at all. But assuming the diabetic traveling man wants to travel and has some destinations lying to the east or west, what are your suggestions on making insulin adjustments?

Dr. Lodewick: I'll make it as simple as possible, but you do have to put a little thought into what you're doing. For an insulin-dependent man who crosses time zones, it may be necessary to slightly reduce or increase his insulin, especially if he is crossing three or more time zones. For stable Type II's on one dose a day, if the flight *lengthens* the day, as it does flying from east to west, a small percentage of extra insulin at the end of the day might help to keep blood sugars down to start the next day at a good level.

For instance, when flying from the east coast to the west coast, the day is 3 hours (or about one-eighth) longer. Also, a small amount of extra snacking or eating may take place. As a result the blood sugar climbs higher from less physical activity plus the extra eating. A Type I on multiple doses of Regular insulin should take about one-eighth (about 10–15%) more insulin at the end of the travel day. The next day, just give yourself the usual doses.

On the trip back from the west coast to the east coast, take about one-eighth (10–15%) *less* insulin because the day is shortened by three hours or one-eighth of the day. On arising the next day, again just take the usual doses.

For Type I's such as myself, who take more than one dose, it's easy. In fact, the more doses a person takes, the easier it is to make the small adjustments in insulin. This is particularly true for those who are on the multiple dose regimen or on insulin pumps using the basal–bolus method of control. For east-to-west travel, a small extra Regular may be used toward the end of the day to cover any extra eating or longer physical inactivity during the longer day. On the way back, a small decrease in the Regular insulin or night-time insulin is probably advisable because of the shorter day.

June and Barbara: The other problem that everyone with diabetes has is getting their bodies to adjust to the new time zone and coping with jet lag. How does jet lag affect a person with diabetes?

Dr. Lodewick: That's easy—the same way it does a person *without* diabetes. Rapidly traveling through time zones can disrupt your body's circadian (24-hour bodily) rhythms and can result in jet lag. Irritability, fatigue, aching muscles, and digestive disorders are common complaints. Some of these, however, are the same symptoms associated with poor diabetes control. To help alleviate jet lag symptoms, cut down on coffee and other caffeine products and drink plenty of water before, during, and after the flight. (There can be as much as one quart of water lost on a three-and-a-half-hour flight because of the dry air circulated at high altitudes.)

Also, make sure your diabetes is not causing the symptoms by not letting it get out of control. To be sure it's *not* your diabetes, monitor your control with blood sugar testing. Then you won't overeat or overdrink, and you'll know that it's not out-of-control diabetes that is mimicking the jet lag symptoms of irritability and fatigue. And you certainly wouldn't want to have a double-dose of these symptoms by having out-of-control diabetes *and* jet lag on top of it.

June and Barbara: Although diabetics get the same symptoms of jet lag as nondiabetics, unfortunately they can't take all the same remedies. Charles F. Ehret and Lynne Walter Scanlon, authors of *Overcoming Jet Lag* (Berkley Books), advocate a special diet starting two to four days before taking off on a time zone change flight. This diet—known as the "Argonne anti jet lag diet"—was developed in experiments at the Argonne National Laboratory in Illinois. The problem with it for diabetics is that it involves alternating days of feasting and fasting. The feast days are high in protein and calories (as much as 1,000 more calories than you would normally consume). The fast days involve high-protein breakfasts and lunches but high-carbohydrate dinners. The total calories on the fast days can be as low as 700. As you can see, this would be inappropriate for a diabetic since you're supposed to keep your diet on a fairly even keel in nutrients, calories, and carbohydrates.

The Argonne National Laboratory and authors Ehret and Scanlon did come up with many other jet lag adjusting techniques that *can* be incorporated into a diabetic traveling man's lifestyle. Here are a selection, with our annotations, of some of the tips we consider most important for diabetics that author Charles Ehret, Ph.D. (Senior Scientist Emeritus at Argonne National Laboratory and President of General Chronobionics Inc., Hinsdale, IL 60521) gave in an article in the *Los Angeles Times.*

1. Leave home well rested, physically strong, and mentally alert, with your body clock strongly set in home time

and your body in the best working order. Avoid extra chores, late night work, last-minute shopping sprees, and endless bon voyage parties. A 15-minute cushion of extra sleep per night before and after your usual eight hours can add to your feeling of well-being if indulged in for three or four nights before a trip.

2. Plan your itinerary carefully; avoid too much zig-zagging across time zones. If you can avoid it, don't arrive at your destination later than midnight, especially during the "circadian pits" (from 2 to 4 A.M.). Try to choose flight schedules that let you arrive after breakfast and before 8:30 at night so that you have time to settle in and enjoy your night's accommodations before it's time to sleep.

3. Travel in comfort. Wear soft, loose-fitting garments and shoes and take along a suitably equipped travel kit. The kit should contain a pair of eye shades and ear plugs to shut out light and noise and a soft pair of slippers to slip on during the flight. The kit should also include a small food reserve containing high-protein granola bars, cheese and crackers, or a small carton of yogurt. High-protein foods are needed because they tend to stimulate the get-up-and-go part of our metabolism. (Note: This food reserve is particularly important for insulin-taking diabetics because you never know when your flight or the food service may be delayed and your insulin will be demanding that you eat when there is nothing available.)

4. Use light to help you make the jet lag adjustment. It's a powerful clock resetter for all living things. For two to four days before and for the first three days after a trip, enjoy plenty of bright light during the day, preferably outdoors. Then be sure that your sleeping quarters are dark at night. If your flight was eastbound, on the day you arrive at your destination, get plenty of outdoor bright light throughout the morning. If you are outdoors in the afternoon, wear sunglasses. If your

flight was westbound, get plenty of outdoor bright light only during the afternoon.

5. Get plenty of exercise daily during the day's active phase and sufficient rest and relaxation during the day's inactive phase. When in flight at destination wake-up time, pace the aisles of the aircraft or do isometric exercises at your seat. When you do reach your destination, do lots of walking before and after each meal.

6. Include deep breathing with your exercise and make a special effort to move lots of oxygen through your lungs. Where space permits, jogging or other aerobic exercise is beneficial. Avoid smoking areas where air pollution levels are high. Oxygen is a powerful clock resetter.

Ehret also recommends that you do *not* use dietary supplements, drugs, and sleeping pills, which are sometimes recommended as jet lag cures. He believes that not only are they not beneficial, but some may have harmful side effects. For diabetics, we double his warning, especially in the case of sleeping pills. You don't want to zonk yourself when you're already disoriented because of jet lag and your body is giving you mixed signals of high and low blood sugar. Sleeping pills are especially hazardous if you're traveling alone with no one to notice if you don't wake up on schedule in the morning.

Even without sleeping pills, many diabetics fear traveling alone. A college professor friend of ours was mourning over the fact that she had no one to travel with who knew anything about diabetes—or who cared to learn. She was envious that June has Barbara to go on trips with and suggested that we start a Rent-A-Barbara service for would-be travelers. Until we get that service going, do you have any tips to make solo travel less disturbing?

Dr. Lodewick: Business travel is tough on a man. It's even tougher than ordinary when the man has to travel alone and there is no companion or spouse to accompany him, as is the case when a pleasure trip is planned. I know myself that when I do travel alone on such occasions, I have to be that much more careful to ensure good control and to spot-check abnormal blood sugars. Although I've not had any problems, it's not as comforting being by myself as it is when my wife Maureen and I travel together. Most diabetic travelers I know who have problems with hypoglycemia tend to let their sugars run a little on the high side to make sure they don't drop below normal range.

In general, though, I'd say that as a solo traveler you should have no major problems and should be able to keep in reasonably good diabetes control. A knowledge of food, how to incorporate some refreshing and healthy exercise into the day's events, proper use of medication (insulin, oral pills, or other medications you may need), and blood sugar testing are essential tools.

June and Barbara: Businessmen or other professionals who attend conferences that last several days would probably appreciate suggestions on how to get some exercise during long-term sedentary periods.

Dr. Lodewick: No matter where you go or where you stay, exercise is always available if you look for it. Many hotels have pools, an increasing number now have gyms, some provide maps with jogging courses marked, and you can always just go out the door and take a long walk. When you're attending conferences, try to swim, jog, or walk before you start the morning sessions. If you can grab a few minutes at lunch time, take a walk around the block or even around the hotel if it's a large complex. In the evening, try for another swim or jog or at least try to walk to dinner and back.

Remember that it's important to take the time out for exercise so you'll always stay fit, feel your best, and function in top form on the trip—and not put on any extra pounds.

June and Barbara: Incidentally, the Fodor people have recently published a book that will help men to stay fit while they travel: *Health and Fitness Vacations*. This is a guide to exercise opportunities in 35 U.S. cities. It focuses on hotel fitness facilities, health clubs that allow walk-ins, the best running routes, where to rent and ride bicycles, where to play golf and tennis, and even conveniently located sports supply stores in case you forgot some important piece of sports clothing or equipment. So now there are no excuses for not getting your exercise on business trips.

Along with worrying about how to get exercise, many diabetics are concerned about having to eat all their meals out when they're on a trip. One basic rule we recommend is to make sure the restaurant is open by calling ahead. We've learned this from all the times we've gone clear across town to a special restaurant that was recommended in a guide book only to find that 1) it's not open that night or 2) it's closed to the public because they're having a private party or 3) the whole place has been bulldozed and is now a parking lot or has been replaced with a high rise or 4) the cuisine has drastically changed. Once in Paris we took a long Metro trip to a recommended bistro called *Aux Bonnes Choses* only to find that it had turned into *Aux Bonnes Choses de Viet-Nam* with a menu of Vietnamese dishes written in French which was beyond our poor powers to translate. Since June had already taken her insulin, we had to eat at the first place we found where we could understand the menu. The restaurant was so bad that no one was in it except a priest, who was probably only there because he was having a free dinner. This sort of problem can be avoided with a call to the restaurant. It's also a good idea to make a reservation if they take them. Restaurants seem to like you better if you make them feel sought-after by reserving a table. And it doesn't hurt to mention that a member of your party has diabetes and needs to be seated promptly. That way you'll be less likely to encounter that old ''your-table-isn't-quite-ready-would-you-like-to-wait-in-the-bar?'' scam.

But let's assume the restaurant is there and functioning and your table is ready. How do you handle the dining out situation?

Dr. Lodewick: It's not all that hard to handle. Dining out in restaurants does not need to be a problem in terms of estimating the approximate number of calories. It is important, however, to be aware that because of poor water purification systems in certain countries, such as in the Far East and Mexico, infectious illness is possible, and learning what food and drinks to avoid is important. Most travel guide books have this information and your travel agent may be able to help with this, too.

Aside from that, rest assured that as long as a man is well versed in the varied calories in foods he should not have a problem because of the foods he eats at a restaurant, unless he overeats. Whether it's eating at McDonald's or a fancier restaurant, he should be able to estimate approximately the number of calories he needs to keep his sugar controlled.

For instance, if I eat out at a romantic restaurant as Maureen and I did this past Valentine's Day, I can keep to my diet and still have a delicious meal. I started with Cocktail de Crevettes (shrimp cocktail, low in carbohydrates), followed by Potage du Jour (cold borscht, very nutritious, into which I dipped my French bread), and Salade Mêlée (mixed salad with vinegar and olive oil, good for my heart). My entrée was broiled swordfish with fresh unbuttered vegetables. Not leaving out dessert, I concluded with a luscious bowl of fresh red raspberries (without the vanilla ice cream). To whet our romantic appetites (that is usually not necessary), we added a glass of Fumé Blanc before and during the meal.

June and Barbara: The meal you selected sounds wonderful. It's true that as long as you know what you're eating and have a basic knowledge of nutrition (which isn't difficult to acquire), you can eat virtually anywhere in the world. We do suggest that before going to a foreign country you study the cookbooks of that culture so you have an idea of what the food contains when you order a meal. For example, had we studied a Vietnamese cookbook written in French, we could have gone right into *Aux Bonnes Choses de Viet-Nam* and had a fine and interesting meal with no problems.

Another thing you might remember while traveling in the United States or abroad is that when you eat out often, it's difficult to get enough fiber in your diet. Barbara—our fiber fanatic—recommends Fiber-Excel or Fiber Supreme to supplement your diet when you travel. Fiber Supreme is particularly good for diabetics because it has fewer carbohydrates than most fiber supplements (only 5 grams per serving) and has an addition of guar gum, which is purported to help lower blood sugar.

But we've been doing all this talking about winging off through time zones; maybe we should come down to earth for a while. More men travel—and travel more often—by automobile than any other way. We always advise Type I diabetics to take their blood sugar before driving even short distances to make sure it's not low, since low blood sugar while driving can make you as much a threat to others and yourself as being drunk while driving. We've known several people who have had accidents while in the throes of hypoglycemia. It's also a good idea to keep Dextrosols and a good collection of snacks in the car when you're on a long trip or if you commute a long way to and from work. You may need these should you be delayed in traffic until past your regular meal time.

Dr. Lodewick: Testing blood sugar before driving is *always* recommended for Type I's. But as a general rule for both Type I's and Type II's, long drives tend to cause *high* blood sugars rather than low. And it's for the same reason that it happens on long airplane flights: immobility. I've observed my own blood sugar go above 300 mg/dl when driving a long distance in a car. It's just like a person who's been hospitalized. His blood sugars may go high even with many fewer calories. For me, as for many others, a cutback in calories under such circumstances is frequently needed.

June and Barbara: On the subject of sitting in cars and driving, we would be remiss if we didn't bring up the subject of the Great American Dream Vacation. This is when you pile the whole family (or at least the wife) and all the luggage into the car at the crack of dawn "to get an early start" and then you drive and drive and drive to try to make 200 or 300 miles before lunch. You eat lunch (looking repeatedly at your watch to make sure you aren't spending too much time eating) and then leap back into the car to try to make another 300 miles before dinner. After dinner you're too tired to do much more than watch a little television and drop off to sleep before 10 o'clock so you can get another early start the next morning. That's pretty much the story of the vacation, punctuated by a few brief stops at an occasional reptile farm or curio shop with a day or two at a theme park. You come back having "made" 6,000 to 7,000 miles. And who knows how many over 200 blood sugars you've also made?

This is, of course, an exaggeration. But there's much truth in it. We've heard similar tales from diabetic women whose husbands have taken them on the Great American Dream Vacations. And we've heard it from women whose diabetic husbands insist on this sort of travel even though it plays havoc with their diabetes control. On top of being unhealthy in the extreme for everyone—diabetic and nondiabetic alike—it's a rotten vacation. About all you see is the world whizzing by in a blur out the car window.

We always recommend taking vacations in which you get as much exercise as possible. Go to just one city and walk every inch of it so that you truly experience it and make it yours forever. We love to do that in San Francisco, including climbing all the hills and walking the Golden Gate Bridge (both directions) for a spectacular view of the city, taking the boat to Alcatraz and walking all over that. There's no end to the walking you can do if you put your mind to it. And when there's no end to the walking you do, there's almost no end to the eating you can do. Eating new foods is one of the most enjoyable aspects of a vacation—one that has to be extremely curtailed if you spend all your time in a sitting position.

Another great thing to do on a vacation is to go somewhere where you can practice a sport you enjoy or take lessons to learn a new one. Not only do you get the exercise from participating in the golf, tennis, skiing, skating, or whatever, you've honed your skills in the sport and can keep using those skills for pleasure, health, and lowering of blood sugar throughout your whole life.

It's not easy to pry yourself out of the car, though, especially if you truly enjoy driving as most men do. One diabetic woman, whose husband had just retired and was celebrating with a Great American Dream Vacation of driving their camper from Pasadena, California, all the way to Alaska, had to resort to desperate measures. Instead of putting their two Irish setters in a kennel for the trip, she convinced her husband to take them along. They, in turn, insisted on getting out and running around for exercise and related activities about every hour. She could then get out and exercise too. She said it was probably the slowest trip anyone ever made to Alaska, and also one of the best. They really saw the territory along the way. They felt good at the end of every day, and her blood sugar stayed in excellent control.

The Great European Dream Vacation is just as detrimental as the Great American one. This is when you get in a bus, car, or train and "see" seven countries in two weeks. There's the same old lack of exercise along with the accompanying lack of being able to eat much of the interesting foreign cuisine and the fact that you hardly experience any of the delights of the countries you go through. Above all, there's the lousy blood sugar control.

When it comes to foreign travel, we advise that you take your "second trip" first. Listen to any person who's just come back from one of those whirlwind multicountry tours. We guarantee their theme will be, "On our next trip, we're just going to Spain" or "Believe me, when I go overseas again, I'm going to only one country and really see it." The first time you go to Europe, it's only human nature to want to hit every country you can. After all, you may never pass that way again. But diabetics need to resist that impulse. Pretend it's your second trip; relax. Be a traveler—not a tourist. Meet people and savor the whole experience. As a diabetic visiting just one country, you can study up on it ahead of time so you'll know what you want to see and do there. Read cookbooks so you know what's in the dishes you'll find in the charming little restaurants you've ferreted out in your guidebook. You can even learn a few pertinent phrases to handle your diabetic emergencies and needs. (*"Ich bin zuckerkrank. Rufen Sie bitte einen Arzt,"* which is German for "I am a diabetic. Please call a doctor"; or *"Io sono diabetico e lo zuccero mi nuoce,"* which is Italian for "I am diabetic and cannot eat anything with sugar in it.") You'll save money by not moving around so much and by understanding the money so you don't get mixed up and pay too much for things.

Maybe you'll have such strength of character that you'll even be able to take your "third trip" to Europe first and go to just one city. We did that once in Rome. We stayed there three weeks, spending one week in Ancient Rome near the Forum, one in Renaissance Rome near the Piazza Navona, and one in modern Rome near the Via Veneto. It was one of the best and healthiest trips we ever took. There was only one small hazard. When we were staying in the Ancient Rome sector and took our after-dinner walk—the better to stabilize June's blood sugar—we didn't realize it but the streets and sidewalks around the Forum were the places of assignation for the Roman men and the ladies of the evening. Since we were walking in that area, it was assumed that we were there to ply our trade. As a result, cars kept pulling up beside us, making us many offers that we *could* refuse—especially since we didn't understand exactly what they were. A diabetic man presumably wouldn't experience such problems in his nocturnal peregrinations (but he might be accosted by the ladies of the evening).

We'd like to finish off our travel tirade with a personal vacation suggestion. When you've been under a lot of business pressure, there's nothing more relaxing than a beach vacation, especially in the tropics, where you can swim and snorkel in the therapeutic, turquoise waters and stroll along seeking sea shells on beaches soft as talcum powder. Aside from being careful not to fry your hide in the midday sun, are there any tips or warnings you have for the would-be beachcomber?

Dr. Lodewick: Strolling along the beach can cause problems if the diabetic's feet are not in healthy condition. I've seen too many cases of blistered feet, some of which subsequently became infected and required partial amputations in diabetic men or women who have walked on very hot sand or sometimes just walked long distances.

This should never happen. Most, if not all, of these people had significant neuropathy, so they could not tell that the sand was hot. Many of them didn't know that they had neuropathy, which rendered them incapable of sensing heat. They could have the same problem with not feeling sharp objects in the sand that could cause a wound. That's why you should insist that your doctor check you for neuropathy. If neuropathy is present, always avoid going barefoot.

June and Barbara: There is even one more way that you must protect your feet, especially when vacationing in the tropics. In areas where there is a lot of coral under water, it is advised that everyone wear plastic or rubber "water shoes" while swimming because a coral cut can easily get infected. This warning goes double for diabetics. These shoes are usually readily obtainable in areas where coral is a problem. But to be on the safe side, pick up a pair at home before leaving. Check with your local sporting goods store. If they don't have any in stock they may be willing to order them for you.

Now that we have everybody geared up and ready to go, do you have any final tips for diabetic men to tuck into their travel bags?

Dr. Lodewick: Yes. Here are some tips that I consider particularly important.

- *Always* have sugar (Dextrosols or other glucose tablets) with you.

- Be careful breaking-in new shoes and don't take new shoes on a trip.

- Wear antiblister socks. (Double Lay-R: 1-800-392-8500).

- If you get sick in a foreign country, contact the American Consulate or an American Express office to find out where to get good medical help.

- If you need a diabetes specialist in a foreign country, contact International Diabetes Association, Brussels, Belgium (telephone: 32-2-647-4414).

- Bring a prescription or letter from your doctor indicating that you need to carry insulin syringes so you won't have trouble with foreign customs—or even American customs when you come home. A diabetes I.D. card and/or identification bracelet is also helpful in avoiding problems.

- You may need immunizations. Check with your local health department and/or doctor to see which ones would be advisable.

- Bring along a record of your current medical condition, especially if you have any special medical problems besides your diabetes.

- Check to see if you have health insurance that covers a hospital stay if an accident occurs away from home or overseas. If not, ask your travel agent if he or she knows of any short-term policy you could take out.

- Write or call ahead to Intermedic for a list of English-speaking doctors in your destination country: 777 Third Avenue, New York, NY 10017 (telephone: 1-212-486-8974).

- Bon voyage.

POSTSCRIPT

Now Voyager

One final bit of travel advice: don't wait too long to do your traveling. We've known people who didn't travel at all during most of their lives because they were "saving it up" until they retired. Then they were going to do Something Significant like take six months or a year to travel around the world. That's like saying you're going to abstain from sex all of your life until you retire and then you're going to have a real orgy.

In the first place, you're deprived of all the mind-expanding and stress-reducing benefits of travel that could enrich your life and enhance your talents. In the second place, travel is a vigorous, sometimes rigorous activity. You need to keep in training for it, gradually building up your traveling skills, learning how to handle all problems and take advantage of all possibilities. The more often you travel, the easier and more pleasurable it gets and the less your diabetes gets in your way—until you hardly know it's there at all.

The
DIABETIC MAN
IN YOUR LIFE
· · · ·
Co-Dependency Takes a Holiday

Co-dependency, the current buzzword and begetter of best-sellers, is a valid concept that has grown in scope and significance over the last few years. At first it was just applied to a person (usually a woman) who was married to an alcoholic and whose ongoing aid, comfort, and covering up abilities "enabled" him to continue in his alcoholism. Later, co-dependency began to embrace the problems experienced by any significant other of a person with any type of addiction. Now, as defined by Melody Beattie, author of two books on co-dependency, it has been broadened to mean being affected by someone else's behavior and obsessed with controlling it.

That definition can apply to almost anyone, but it has special significance for wives, mothers, sisters, daughters, and girlfriends of diabetic men. Not that it can't apply to fathers, brothers, and male friends as well, but as Wendy Kaminer, writing in the *New York Times Book Review*, puts it, "In our culture, women have long been assigned primary responsibility for the family's emotional balance, and co-dependency is often described as a feminine disease (rooted in the model of a co-alcoholic wife, it's commonly associated with compulsive caretaking)."

Anne Wilson Schaef, author of *When Society Becomes an Addict* and *Meditations for Women Who Do Too Much*, calls co-dependency "the disease of people who love too much" and, more bluntly, "the doormat syndrome."

In diabetes we see co-dependency in action all the time. Women come in wringing their hands over a diabetic husband, boyfriend, or son who "won't take care of himself," who "just ignores his diabetes," or who's "going to go blind or have kidney failure or die." "What am I going to do with him?" they ask. They do their best to help by reading every book they can find on the subject of diabetes and turning themselves into lay experts on the subject. They buy blood sugar testing meters and learn how to use them and try to do the testing. They often learn how to give insulin injections and sometimes do all the injecting for the recalcitrant diabetic. These women would gladly test their own blood and take the insulin themselves if it would be possible to do so and let the diabetic man off the hook.

The sad thing is we often see the same women over and over again still telling the same story. No matter how much they learn or how hard they try, the diabetic man continues doing just exactly what he wants to, which is having as little as possible to do with his diabetes therapy. If the two people involved here are engaged in this sort of tug-of-war and manipulation, then all the co-dependency definitions fit.

This certainly doesn't mean that a woman shouldn't learn all she can about diabetes and help a diabetic man control his disease. If you're helping and it makes you feel happy and loving and it makes him feel happy and loved, and if his diabetes is in good control and getting better, then it's great! This is the way life should be. It's working for everyone involved.

But if it's *not* working, if he's abdicating all responsibility for his diabetes and feeling angry and resentful toward you for the efforts you're putting forth to try to keep him healthy, if you're turning into a frazzled, despairing nag, then it's *not* the way life should be. Changes need to be made. "Right," you may say, "changes *do* need to be made. He needs to get his diabetic act together."

True, he does, but he may never get it together if you devote your every conscious moment to trying to get it together for him. As Jacqueline Castine says in her book, *Recovery from Rescuing*, "Helping is most effective when it empowers the other person to help himself. We frequently help others because we see them as helpless. It's no wonder that they become angry instead of grateful." She also emphasizes that you should "not try to control and change his actions, but through under-standing and awareness to change [your own] reactions." You should, she succinctly puts it, "love and let be." Put the accent on the love part. You don't finally furiously throw down the syringe or the Exchange Lists and shout, "The hell with you. You can take care of your own damned diabetes. I don't care anymore. I give up." No, you just quietly and firmly but *lovingly* hand over his diabetes to him. Let him become responsible for his own actions and his own decisions, and if necessary, let him suffer the consequences. That's the tough part of tough love. True, he may not accept his diabetes and take charge, but neither will he if you continue to fret over him and badger him.

If you are able to hand over his diabetes to him, a strange phenomenon may occur. Recovered co-dependents often tell the same story. When, after years of struggle and defeat, they gave up trying to control the other person, that person decided to take charge of himself.

We heard of a similar situation from a diabetic man named Paul who was diagnosed diabetic at the age of ten. Part of his denial was an absolute refusal to learn to give himself insulin injections. His mother had to give them to him. One week his aunt, who was a nurse, came for a visit. When she saw what was going on, she was aghast. "You're not always going to be around when Paul needs to take insulin," she told her sister. "He's going to have to do it himself and he's going to have to do it right now." With that she sat Paul down and told him that he'd better learn how to give himself injections because nobody else was going to do it for him anymore. When Paul violently and vociferously demurred, the aunt said, "Fine. You don't have to give yourself an injection if you don't want to, but if you don't, you'll be dead in three days." Paul's hysterical tears dried on his face. He learned to give himself the injections and has continued to give them to himself over the 28 years since.

Now all this tough love and giving up of control isn't easy, especially for a high-octane, guilt-powered, compulsive caretaker. To give yourself strength and resolve, you may need to read a few dozen of the innumerable co-dependency self-help books currently on the market. You may need to join or start a support group for parents, wives, sisters, or girlfriends of diabetics. (As far as we know, there's no Diabet-Anon, but there should be!) You may even have to seek psychological counseling for yourself or group therapy for your family. Then, finally, if all your strenuous efforts in second-hand diabetes control fail, it's worth trying what the Buddhists call "effortless effort."

Jacqueline Castine uses this quotation from *The Way of Life According to Lao-tzu* as the epigraph for her book. You might use it as the epigraph for the rest of your life with a diabetic man.

If I keep from meddling with other people,
  they take care of themselves,
If I keep from commanding other people,
  they behave themselves,
If I keep from preaching at people,
  they improve themselves...
                    —*June and Barbara*

WHAT YOU'LL FIND HERE

SECRECY

CONFLICT

COOKING FOR A DIABETIC

SQUEAMISHNESS AND FEAR OF DIABETES THERAPIES

DEALING WITH HYPOGLYCEMIA

CHILDREN'S PERCEPTIONS OF FATHER'S DIABETES

ADVANTAGES OF DIABETES

RESENTMENT

COPING

Note: The following questions evolved from our conversations with people who love and who are valiantly trying to help the diabetic man in their lives. The answers are real-life solutions that we, Dr. Lodewick, or others who are involved with a diabetic man have worked out, usually through trial and error. (You have to expect errors and try, try, again!)

What can I do if my man won't even discuss his diabetes with me and totally declines my help?

June and Barbara: We don't know exactly what your particular situation is, but we can assure you that the masculine tendency to hide diabetes is sometimes carried to such extremes that it's almost impossible to believe. One of our male diabetic friends admitted to us that he was married for two years before he confessed to his wife that he had diabetes. We not only wonder why he would want to do such a thing but also how he managed it. The following letter we received shows a classic example of this masculine denial phenomenon and what one woman did to cope with it.

Dear June and Barbara:

I am not a diabetic but began going with one a few months ago. Only in conversation with some others did he admit he was a diabetic and then said no more about it—and only because I accidentally came across his needle and insulin did I realize I knew NOTHING about diabetes. It really hit me, so without his knowledge I began reading every book I could find (yours were the best for giving really heart-of-the-matter information) and am starting a five-week Tuesday night course given by a local hospital. He knows I've signed up but has still made no comment!

We may try living together this summer, and whether he ever says anything about his diabetes or not, I need to know all I can to help care for him. It's frustrating to *guess* at things, but it's all I can do for now. He hates to be hounded or fussed over.... Maybe in time he'll "let me in."

I really never realized how much there was to diabetes until I started reading. I am impressed with my friend's control of it, because for two months I didn't have a clue. I thought his use of artificial sweeteners and refusal of cakes was only a diet or health-food regime! But, talk about lonely, try wanting to help someone you care about and not being able to because he won't ever talk about it. I don't know how long it's been since he was diagnosed, what kind of insulin he uses (I peeked at the bottle; it's French, as he's here from overseas for research), how often he uses it, where he keeps glucagon, or even if he has any (do they do it differently in Europe?). I have begun carrying in my purse Monojel for insulin reactions,

packets of honey and sugar, Lifesavers, one can each
of orange and grape juice, and glucose tablets. (Information I got from your exercise book.) I don't know
what else to do. The hospital course, I hope, will include
lessons on how to inject, how to handle emergencies,
and so forth.

All I can do is learn everything and hope I can do
one of them right whenever it's needed.

THANKS!!!

This woman's anguish really leaps out at you from the
page. We think her course of action is very sound. Educating
yourself in diabetes is the most comforting (to yourself) and
helpful (to him) thing you can do. We can only hope that this
man is eventually able to overcome his emotional barrier and
confide in this woman. If not, we fear that the relationship can't
last. What relationship could under those circumstances?

Another tactic some women use with success is to read
books and, when they find a good one, try to get the man to
read it. Sometimes it works and sometimes it doesn't. Here's a
letter from a girl who met with success and wrote to tell us
about it.

Dear June and Barbara:

In my attempt to learn more about how to help
my fiancé control his diabetes I recently found *The
Peripatetic Diabetic* at the library. In my reading of it
I stopped several times to read him funny parts. He
was amused (first time *ever* I've seen him laugh at
diabetes) and asked to read the book. He has now
taken it on a business trip and I get comments on
what he's read each day by phone. What an "upper"!
I believe we're (he's) on a positive new track mentally
and thank you, thank you, thank you!

How can I deal with a husband who just argues with me when I try to get him to improve his poor diabetes care and who even seems to go out of his way to do the wrong thing?

Dr. Lodewick: Most men I know prefer to take charge of their own condition, without having to be told how to do it. If they do the right thing, all the better. But if they do the wrong thing, the responsibility is theirs, and theirs alone. The only problem is that the wrong thing may hurt the entire family, not just themselves. But with diabetes especially, the wrong thing is more often than not done out of ignorance and because they just don't realize the connection between their bad habits and their poor control. This is the same male invulnerability myth we've discussed before.

The problem arises in marriage when husbands don't listen to their wives and the wives begin to nag. And besides, who likes to be told what he should be doing? Constant nagging only makes the situation worse. If you nag and nag and get no response, or worse, your man goes out of his way to do the wrong thing, STOP NAGGING. Instead, be sympathetic and supportive. Help him learn more about diabetes care. Good diabetes education makes everyone feel less helpless. One 18-year-old young man refused to take insulin despite his physician's advice. Only when he learned that insulin would allow him to eat more and develop an enviable physique did he agree to use it. Subsequently, he had no problem taking insulin, especially when he saw the results.

The goal is to make your husband (or son or friend) realize that with proper knowledge of the basics of diabetes care, his life can be perfectly normal. You might try making a contract with him. Promise that you will stop nagging, commanding, and preaching when he proves that he is caring for himself or gives a legitimate reason why he is not. The reward of a nonnagging wife may be just the goad a man needs to change his self-destructive ways.

Unfortunately, there are men who will not take care of themselves, even when they know the possible consequences. Some of these men are gamblers; they are gambling that overeating or overdrinking and poor diabetes control will not cause *them* problems. In other words, they are fully aware of what can happen to them, but they refuse to believe it. They are willing to take the risk. These men will not even come to the doctor until complications strike them.

There are other men who suffer from depression, who seem to have lost the joy of living. This adversely affects their family, friends, and job. They may be knowledgeable about diabetes, but they just don't care. These men need to realize that they are having a negative effect not only on themselves but also on their loved ones. Upon realizing that they are doing this, they may agree to psychiatric treatment and even the use of medication to alleviate their depression and regain their zest for living. Only then will they be motivated to take control of their diabetes.

Since I do most of the grocery shopping and cooking for my family, now that my husband is diabetic, am I going to have to start buying and cooking differently?

June and Barbara: You probably are, and it will be good for everyone concerned. As we have emphasized, the so-called diabetic diet is the one we should all be eating, but it sometimes takes a diagnosis of diabetes in a family member to provide the impetus for us to do it. The clue here is to make the changes gradually. Don't try to switch overnight from hot dogs, french fries, and hot fudge sundaes to steamed broccoli, skinless poached chicken, and canned pears packed in water. The chorus of "Yuck!" will be deafening, and your dietary improvement program will die aborning.

In fact, you may never serve your family broccoli, and skinless poached chicken, and canned pears packed in water—if these are not popular favorites around your dinner table. Yet you may still be able to serve perfect meals for diabetes and general family health. As former writers for such magazines as *Gourmet* and *Bon Appétit* and as "foodies" who avidly seek out interesting dishes in restaurants at home and in travel, we would *never* serve or eat a meal that is diabetically appropriate but boring and "yucky." With a diabetic diet it's easy to have it both ways—healthy and deliciously exciting.

To get started, you should buy yourself a good diabetes cookbook. The recipes in it will include nutritional information, including diabetes exchanges, that will allow you to serve your husband the right amount for his prescribed diet. There are many diabetes cookbooks now available at most bookstores, and some from the American Diabetes Association are available at your local chapter.

Pick out some recipes from your diabetic cookbook that are closest to the dishes your family already likes and start with those. They may not even be aware that the household menu has changed for the better. Next, gradually add new dishes that sound interesting to you. Then get more adventuresome. When you go out to a restaurant and have something the family particularly enjoys, try to duplicate it at home in an even more healthy style with no sugar, low salt, and low fat (and try to use vegetable, not animal, fat). Use as many fresh fruits and vegetables as you can. You may even start a garden and grow your own. Gardening is a great family activity, it's good exercise for the diabetic member, and your harvest will taste a zillion times better than anything you can get in the market. In other words, take the dietary changes necessary for diabetes and make them into a Great Dining Adventure for the whole family—including yourself.

But even if you don't want to go all that far into gastronomic outer space, following the diabetic diet at home isn't that hard, as Dr. Lodewick's wife, Maureen, points out:

> Many people wonder how I manage to help my husband with his diet while satisfying my four children at the same time. The truth is, Pete has no special diet. The family all enjoys the same

diet—one that is very nutritious and healthy. In fact, our kids have come home astonished at all the junk food found in their friends' houses. I can't say that we are dietary puritans, for I must confess that my children and I adore ice cream, which Pete is sometimes embarrassed to go out and pick up for us. He's afraid of setting a bad example for any of his patients who might see him buying it. I'm sure they could understand that it was for his wife and four healthy children!

Perhaps we should see if Dr. Lodewick has some suggestions on the diabetic diet both as one who follows it and as one who tries to get patients to follow it.

Dr. Lodewick: I believe a good husband–wife relationship is one of the primary ingredients in healthy, appetizing, and diabetically appropriate menus. I think this is illustrated in the following story.

THE CASE OF THE DISGRUNTLED HUSBAND AND HIS DIET

Ralph, a long-term patient of mine, failed to get good control of his diabetes, but he only accepted partial responsibility for this. Although he agreed that he, himself, was the one who was guilty of overeating, he placed part of the blame on his wife. "As far as my special diet is concerned, she couldn't care less," he complained. "She cooks for everyone else in the family, and she's not about to make a special effort to cook for me. So if she cooks an overabundance of food, I am going to eat it. I know I have to take control, but when the food is in front of me, I have a hard time. I have a hard time even asking her the time of day, let alone to cook a special meal."

This man has nearly an unsolvable problem unless his wife does start making a special effort (or he divorces her, which I'm not advocating). Possibly he could make her a little more inclined to help him get the right food by putting some romance back into the marriage. He could send her flowers and take her out and do other things that would lift up her spirits. Then she might become more interested in providing the appropriate meals.

I can very much identify with this man's plight. Fortunately, my wife, Maureen, does make a special effort to provide nutritionally healthy meals for me—although she's not perfect, either. Occasionally, she will even have ice cream in the house. Sometimes she makes me go out to buy it for her and our children. Ice cream, an all-time Lodewick favorite well before I got diabetes, is definitely a temptation for me. Although a limited amount of ice cream is all right for most people with diabetes and will not raise the blood sugar, I must confess that I am guilty of the same sin as my patient just described. I will often eat more than prescribed, especially if it's Häagen-Dazs butter pecan and it's staring me in the face. So my advice is, if you really want to help the diabetic man in you life, don't tempt him. (I mean, of course, don't tempt him by keeping his favorite forbidden food around the house. Other temptations are always welcome!)

On the other hand, if you can keep healthy snack foods, soup with beans, fresh fruit and vegetables, and other healthy but tasty foods on hand for the diabetic man in your life, it will go a long way toward helping him keep his blood sugar controlled.

June and Barbara: You can see from this Rashomon-like tale of ice cream in the Lodewick household that even learned diabetes specialists and their wives experience some of the same frustrations and minor misunderstandings with the diabetic diet that amateurs do. But love and a sense of humor and honest communication will conquer all.

How can I keep other people from acting so frightened and squeamish when my son (or husband) tests his blood sugar or takes a shot?

June and Barbara: Squeamishness is a real problem. There are people who get nauseated and/or hysterical over anything to do with blood or needles. Try this passage from Sue Grafton's *"F" Is for Fugitive*. In it, the detective heroine, Kinsey Millhone, describes looking after an elderly diabetic woman named Ori for a while until the housekeeper arrives.

> Ori was sitting up in bed, fussing with the ties on her gown. Paraphernalia on the night table and the faint scent of alcohol indicated that Ann had done Ori's glucose test and had already administered her morning dose of insulin. The trace of blood streaked on the reagent strip had dried to a rusty brown. Old adhesive tape was knotted up on the bed tray like a wad of chewing gum. Stuck to it was a cotton ball with a linty-looking dot of red. This before breakfast. Mentally, I could feel my eyes cross, but I bustled about in my best imitation of a visiting nurse. I was accustomed, from long experience, to steeling myself to the sight of violent death, but this residue of diabetic odds and ends nearly made my stomach heave.
>
> (Quoted with permission from Sue Grafton, *F Is for Fugitive*, New York, Henry Holt and Company, Inc., copyright © 1989 by Sue Grafton)

This squeamishness doesn't just exist in fiction. It can happen in real life, as this letter we received from a woman who had just started taking insulin and was using a jet injector, well illustrates.

> Dear June and Barbara:
>   I was having lunch with a friend at a restaurant. We placed our order and I excused myself to go to the ladies' room to take my small amount of insulin. The private toilet stalls were extremely dark, so I waited until the room cleared and then I began to fill the injector. While I was doing this, a woman came in and I was not in a position to stop what I was doing so I continued. After I pushed the button, I was subjected to the greatest tirade I think I've ever heard. It rather boiled down to "you people shouldn't be allowed in

public." I was also told that she had many friends who were diabetic, "and they all take oral insulin."

I managed to remain calm and told her that I'd really love to know where her friends got oral insulin, since my doctor, a specialist in the field, would like to know as much as I would like to know. I guess that having been so shaken by her experience of having to witness such terror left her unable to return to her table at once, and I was able to point out that there was no such thing as "oral insulin" available as yet for diabetics and that her friends were taking oral medications to shock the pancreas into greater production. I also pointed out that I had noticed that she took several pills while I was placing my order, and that she did not leave the table. At that moment I decided it was the last time that I would seek the privacy of a restroom, that if it's socially acceptable to take a pill in public, it is equally as acceptable to take insulin in public, and I have done so ever since.

Fortunately, most people don't react (or overreact) the way Sue Grafton's heroine and the woman in the restroom did. As one friend of a diabetic told us,

Most of our friends are interested in the way Jack tests his blood and gives himself his shots. In the beginning, my family asked him not to check his blood or give himself shots in front of them because it bothered them. (Funny it never bothered me.) Now he does check his blood in front of them and they seem to accept it. He still leaves the room to take his shot, though.

As far as Dr. Lodewick's son Matt is concerned, there's never been any problem in this area.

My friends don't seem to recognize Dad's diabetes. I guess the only evidence to them of his disease is his insulin shots and our family screaming at him to take some sugar because he seems a little low during the annual marathon tennis matches he endures up in the Adirondacks. But still, my dad's acrobatic footwork is a constant reminder to them that diabetes doesn't make him any less of a man.

Years ago when the SugarFree Center was sharing quarters with a construction company, we had some conflict with our building-mates. Although they had a perfectly good phone intercom system, rather than use it, they constantly shouted to one another loudly and profanely. Many of them were also chain smokers and filled the air with their poisonous vapors. As you can imagine, neither of these activities was compatible with trying to teach blood sugar testing to people who were already nervous and disturbed.

When we protested about what they were doing, they countered that they didn't like what we were doing either. "Sticking people's fingers and playing around with their blood. It's disgusting!" Fortunately, they moved out a few months later.

Naturally, a diabetic man doesn't need to go out of his way to offend others who are squeamish about needles and blood—and hardly any of them ever do. (In fact, men usually err on the side of being too secretive about it.) A diabetic man should, however, feel perfectly free to do whatever is needed to take care of his diabetes whenever he needs to. June has injected her insulin just about everywhere—including on a bus stop bench in Paris with the Parisians staring in either amazement or revulsion, depending on their personal views of the matter. In airplanes we always explain to our seat mates what June's going to do so they can look away if it bothers them. On the other hand, taking a blood sugar test is such a discreet activity that hardly anyone is offended by it since no one is usually aware that it's happening. This is especially true with the new small meters that look like minicalculators. There's even a new blood-letting device called the Autolet Lite that looks almost identical to a cigarette lighter. Actually, these days a man would probably offend more people who think he's about to light a cigarette than he would people who'd be bothered by a minute drop of blood.

You should, however, encourage the diabetic man to not leave used syringes, cotton, and tissues lying around with blood on them. In this age of AIDS and hepatitis, this is understandably frightening even to people who are not squeamish about needles and blood. Needles are a particular hazard if there are children in the house. And since so much testing and injecting is done in cars in this hurried world, you should be sure he has a trash bag there to collect all the diabetes detritus.

But what if the squeamish person is you, the diabetic man's loved one? What if *you* are profoundly disturbed by the sight or even the thought of blood or a needle going into human flesh—especially dearly beloved human flesh? Well, you're just going to have to tough it out and get over it, just the way a diabetic person who is terrified of needles and blood has to get over it. Be around as often as you can when he tests and takes his injection, and if he doesn't object, watch. After you become inured to the sight, ask him to take your blood sugar from time to time. When that doesn't bother you anymore, have him show you how to test yourself and do that often enough so you feel comfortable doing it.

Finally, if you're a real sport, take a syringe and inject yourself with saline solution. Do it as many times as you need to drive away any feelings of fear and loathing. When you've gradually worked your way through the whole diabetic routine, your squeamishness will be gone forever. Guaranteed. You also will be more capable of helping the diabetic man in your life if he's ever sick and needs someone to test his blood sugar or give him an injection. Even more important, you'll know how to inject glucagon, should he ever pass out from an insulin reaction.

Besides being able to help the diabetic in your life, overcoming this squeamishness (which may really be more of a fear of doing something you've never done before) will give you a great feeling about yourself as a strong and competent person. Enjoy that feeling. You deserve it!

I'm terribly disturbed when my husband starts getting low blood sugar. I seem to fall apart over it more than he does. I'm always afraid that I'll do the wrong thing when I try to help. How can I get over that?

June and Barbara: Sometimes it just takes time. Even Maureen Lodewick—who's a nurse and even had a grandmother with diabetes—had problems dealing with Dr. Lodewick's low blood sugar at first.

> I was initially frightened by the first few episodes of hypoglycemia. As time passed, though, Pete became very conscientious about testing his sugar levels and managed well at balancing his insulin, diet, and exercise so his low blood sugar incidents became fewer and farther between. Still, I know the warning indications and am prepared to assist my husband at a moment's notice with a soda on the tennis court or a glass of orange juice at night.
>
> I recall one night when Pete's sugar had dropped and I was about to go get him some juice, when he asked, "How about making that a roast beef sandwich?" To which I replied, "Get it yourself!" Lest you think me unsympathetic, from past experience I knew that if he was well enough to ask for a roast beef sandwich, he was capable of making it himself. Also at the time I was near exhaustion from taking care of three young children who had managed to simultaneously develop chicken pox!

Maureen is right that you need to become familiar with the warning signals of your man's hypoglycemia. You also have to be familiar with his normal behavior so that you can distinguish between hypoglycemia and his personality quirks. As Maureen says, "When Pete is acting vague or 'spacy,' we usually know that it's not an episode of hypoglycemia. It's just his typical absentminded nature."

When it really *is* hypoglycemia, be prepared by keeping glucose tablets or other blood sugar raisers such as Glutose or Insta-Glucose handy and by learning how to inject glucagon (see Appendix E) in case he has a serious low blood sugar incident and either becomes unconscious or incapable of swallowing. You should also be sure to always keep the glucagon in the same place and *know for sure where that place is* because if you ever have to use it, you're bound to be in a flap and it will be easy to forget where you put it if it's not drilled into your mind.

Do you think the fact that they have a diabetic father will disturb our children or make them feel insecure or fearful that he may die?

June and Barbara: According to Dr. Lodewick's son, Matt, there should be no problem.

As a child, I really can't say that I was aware of diabetes as a life-threatening or even a handicapping disease. My father did everything every other father did, and he always ran around and played with us. As for sports, as I'm sure you've been informed, my dad excelled in them.

My observations of my father, when I was young, did not lead to the belief that diabetes really affected his life. There were times when I recognized the symptoms of diabetes, but even these didn't seem to frighten me about my father's state. For instance, my father's blood sugar would run low and he would, to my eyes, be acting "weird and silly," but I knew that he would return to his normal self shortly with the help of some sugar from orange juice or the like.

By the time I was old enough to be able to think about it, my dad managed his diabetes so well so that it was hard for me to grasp the severity of the disease. As I grew older, though, I learned more about it through researching it and reading articles about it. I began to become confused because I couldn't connect this diabetes I read about with my father. Certainly he didn't seem to have been handicapped by this "serious" disease.

My father has taught me a lot about diabetes, and now I can understand the ill effects of diabetes and how to prevent them. My father also takes excellent care of himself, and to me at least, it seems as if this necessary care doesn't consume much of his time and thus he is able to lead a normal life. So in this way, I am happy that he has diabetes rather than some other serious disease by which his lifestyle truly would be impeded.

This shows that when the father takes good care of himself and is matter-of-fact about his diabetes, the children can adjust beautifully and develop an understanding and acceptance of the disease and not be filled with fear and dread over it.

On the other hand, consider this excerpt from the introduction to *The Diabetic Woman*, in which diabetic endocrinologist Lois Jovanovic-Peterson describes the impact her father's diabetes had on her.

> My father had Type I diabetes. By the time he had children, he was already riddled with problems. I remember his morning ritual of testing his urine—with a tablet, which I now know was Clinitest. The test tube became very hot, and the contents then turned an ugly brown or orange. Now I realize that he never, never was in good control. He took his insulin with a glass syringe, which mother boiled. Every afternoon he had an insulin reaction...and if we didn't rush home from school to give him dinner, he was in diabetic coma.
>
> From my earliest memories, Daddy was bedridden and blind. At the time of his death, I was 12; he was 50 with 20 years of diabetes. I promised at his graveside that I would devote my life to curing diabetes.

Dr. Jovanovic-Peterson's father had diabetes back in the days when good control was extremely difficult if not impossible. As you can see from the urine test he was taking, the far more accurate blood sugar testing was not yet available to the individual diabetic. The devastating results of his poor diabetes therapy were horrifying to his young and loving daughter, so much so that when she herself was diagnosed diabetic while in her medical residency (at almost the same age her father had been when he was diagnosed), she went into a complete and almost hysterical state of denial. The idea of having diabetes was too terrible for her to accept.

Today, the choice of good or poor control is up to the individual. The knowledge and tools are there for him to use if he wants to. If he chooses not to use them, not only is he damaging himself and shortening his life, he is indeed blighting the childhood and the later lives of his children, especially if they should someday develop diabetes themselves. Many men who refuse to take care of their diabetes for their own sakes may change if they realize what they're putting their children through. If you're trying to help such a man, perhaps this is the direction for you to take. You might even have him read this section—or if he refuses, read it to him!

Are there any advantages of having a diabetic man in my life?

June and Barbara: We must confess that we made this question up ourselves, since you might never think of asking it and neither would any other person involved with a diabetic man. On the surface it would appear that his diabetes is nothing but negative. But in real life, almost nothing is a total negative, and that includes diabetes. Here's what Matt Lodewick learned from his father's diabetes.

> My father's diabetes has had an impact on my life in several ways, but most significantly on my own health and health care. I feel I have benefited greatly in regard to my diet. If my father didn't have to worry about his intake of foods, then I think I would eat less carefully. Furthermore, I recognize the healthiness of exercise and its effects on the body. Thus, in a kind of stoic way, his diabetes has been very helpful to me, as those things that a diabetic should do in order to maintain good control are the same things that nondiabetics should do to obtain better health.
>
> My father's diabetes has also given me greater compassion for disabled and ill people. I am better able to recognize the struggle that they go through in order to conquer handicaps, and I'm inspired by the greatness of a human's inner strength. It seems natural for me to want to help people in that struggle and

to study medicine as I am now doing. I know my father's diabetes is in great part responsible for my decision to become a doctor myself.

The friend of a diabetic man agrees in many ways with Matt's assessment.

> Bill's diabetes has helped me to change in a lot of ways. One, for instance, is stopping smoking and walking more to get exercise. We even walked in the American Diabetes Association walk-a-thon, or, rather, I walked for the two of us because his mother was very ill and he had to be out of town on the day of the event. We collected the most money of anyone that day for the ADA. Without his diabetes I would never have participated in this event, which was good for both my body and soul.

Diabetes *is* an education. If you really get involved with it, you'll learn a lot that can be as important for you to know as it is for the diabetic man. Besides learning how to improve your own health, the knowledge about diabetes you gain may well help you in certain areas of your professional life, as it did one policeman whose best friend was diagnosed diabetic. "My attitude towards diabetes as a police officer has changed in that I know more now than I ever knew before about the disease."

The following letter, sent to the Captain (and Commanding Officer) of his precinct demonstrates how his new knowledge and attitude improved his performance as a police officer.

> Dear Sir:
>
> May I commend to you in the highest terms, the following two police officers: _____ and _____ [names deleted]. On November 11, being from out-of-town, I was not able to locate where I had parked my car. I roamed the streets of the area in excess of two hours without success. Furthermore, I am a diabetic and needed my insulin dosage, which naturally was at home. I proceeded to the police station for help and was assisted by the above-mentioned two police

officers. These two gentlemen were compassionate, warm, and patiently drove me around until my car was located. Furthermore, Police Officer _____ [the friend of the diabetic] was very knowledgeable about diabetes and was all the more supportive. From the bottom of my heart, I wish to thank you for having these two outstanding officers on your force.

Very truly yours, _____

The police officer with the diabetic friend went on to say that, "Now when a job comes in and the person has diabetes, I listen more carefully to see if it's in my beat and I am not so afraid to handle the job because of my experience with my friend." Incidentally, this police officer recently received a significant promotion. It wouldn't be surprising if his understanding of diabetes contributed to the outstanding performance that caused him to be recognized on the force as a man worthy of rising in the ranks.

We recently heard of another occurrence in which a person's knowledge of diabetes saved the day. This one took place on an airline. As anyone who travels these days is painfully aware, you never know if and when your plane will leave or to where it might be diverted. The time of food service is another great mystery. A diabetic friend of ours, valiantly trying to fly from New York to Las Vegas, had been shunted to a few surprise cities en route. Because of the ups and downs of this particular flight, no meals had been served. His dinner was long overdue. A flight attendant made the announcement that although the next scheduled stop should be Denver, they were actually going to land in Colorado Springs, where they would be on the ground for an hour and passengers would be allowed to deplane and walk around. "Great!" thought our friend. "I'll take my shot and grab something to eat at the airport." He took a little more than his usual dose of insulin because, strapped into his seat all day, he had been so inactive.

The plane landed and he started unbuckling his seat belt, the better to race down the aisle and be first in line at the food concession. But not so fast! The announcement came on that plans had been changed and they would be on the ground for only five minutes and *nobody was allowed to leave the plane.* Our friend is a man to be reckoned with—especially when he's hungry and full of insulin. He marched up to the head flight attendant and started protesting in no uncertain terms that he'd just taken his insulin and he had to get off the plane and find some food. The attendant was obdurate. He certainly couldn't get off the plane. It was going to be taking off almost momentarily, he'd miss the flight, and regulations did not permit his exiting the plane. Our friend continued his protest in increasingly loud and firm terms. The captain emerged from the cabin to see what was going on. When he understood the situation, he ordered the attendant to "let that man off to get some food. We'll hold the plane for him." It turned out the captain had an insulin-taking diabetic daughter.

As Matt Lodewick has pointed out, one of your most valuable gains is the compassion and understanding you develop for other diabetics—indeed for all people with a disease or physical problem. You'll realize from your experience that each of these people is a human being, not just the disease or the physical problem. (You'll never be like some callous hospital personnel who've been known to refer to "the gallbladder in Room 134B" or the "fractured hip in Room 185A.")

You'll also begin to learn the valuable lesson of strength and forbearance in the face of adversity, a lesson that we all inevitably must learn as we face our own life problems.

How can I get rid of my feelings of resentment about diabetes?

June and Barbara: You probably can't unless you're a saint—and there aren't many of those around these days. After all, you have much to be resentful about. It's terribly unfair that your diabetic man or boy should have this intrusive and disruptive disease, so you resent the disease itself and what it's doing to his life. And let's face it, you also resent how it intrudes on and disrupts *your* life. You know something important and disruptive is about to happen from the moment of the diagnosis. As one close friend of a diabetic man wrote us:

> When I first learned that Mike was diagnosed as having diabetes, I never realized the complications he was going to experience both physically and mentally. There was some diabetes in my family, but I never lived with it myself or had any idea of what I was in for. I still remember the Friday back in May 1989 when Mike came home with test strips for urine. I thought he was nuts, but he told me his mother, who is a nurse, told him to use these strips to find out if he might have diabetes. We both did the test several times. His kept turning dark green and mine stayed yellow. We knew then that our lives were going to change.

Obviously you resent it if he doesn't take care of himself and keep his diabetes in control. But you also resent it if he seems to go overboard about it and sometimes even if he just does what he has to do as a diabetic. Does any of this sound familiar?

> Dan's extremely careful with his diet and exercise to the point of being obsessive. He's not kidding about the amount of carbohydrates, protein, fat, and calories he puts into his body.... I resent that sometimes I have to wait for Dan to check his blood sugar—which he seems to always be doing—or take a shot before dinner.... Often my schedule has to change for Dan and it doesn't seem fair.... I sometimes feel frustrated, for instance, having to eat when he does instead of when I want to or, even worse, not being able to eat when I want to because his blood sugar is high and we have to wait for it to come down.

Your feelings are further complicated by the fact that you know he's experiencing the same feelings in reverse. "I feel that he gets frustrated when he sees me get upset about his diabetes."

And on top of everything else, you both feel guilty. He feels guilty that his diabetes is impinging on your life, slowing you down, keeping you from doing what you want to do when you want to do it. And you feel guilty that you resent how his diabetes disrupts your life and your relationship. You know he can't help having diabetes and can't help having to take care of it. You can't blame him—and yet, in a sense, you do. More guilt!

Resentment and guilt, guilt and resentment. Two more negative emotions it would be hard to find and there you both are, constantly wrestling with them every day.

What to do? Again, you need to find acceptance. But it's not just accepting the fact of the disease, but also accepting your feelings about it, realizing that everyone in a close relationship with a diabetic sometimes gets angry, frustrated, and resentful. It doesn't make you a bad person when you behave the way any normal human being would in a similar situation. It doesn't even make you a bad person if you occasionally lose your temper when he's blowing up at you because he has low blood sugar and you can't make him do anything about it. It's an emotional reaction almost as natural and uncontrollable as the reflex that makes you kick when the doctor hits your knee with a hammer. Accept it without assigning blame to yourself.

Of course, if these negative emotions are overwhelming you and undermining your relationship with him, some psychological counseling would certainly be in order. After all, diabetes is forever, and you need to come to terms with it and with your reaction to it just as much as he does.

The important thing for you to do as you daily slog your way through all the muck and mire of diabetes is to try to keep it in perspective. On the wall of our office, we have a motto written on a giant yellow tablet.

> *Don't sweat the small stuff!*
> *P.S. It's all small stuff.*

You might like to hang a copy of that on the wall of your mind.

POSTSCRIPT
Develop a Sixth Sense

In talking to and corresponding with family members and friends of diabetic men, we find that, aside from love, which is a given, there is one indispensable element, one essential mind-set that can make the most difference between success and failure: a sense of humor. Over and over we hear this from people, for example, from Matt Lodewick:

> I learned a great quote that I plan to keep in mind as I live and die and that is—"You've got to look at things hilariously, because they are." This really helps. For as bad as things get, they can be taken humorously also. You can get down when things seem not to be going in the right direction, but that only sends you further into the dark. If, instead of getting down on the situation, you can handle it with a dose of humor, it is only to your advantage. There are so many things you can get down about. You don't even have to look that hard, but I think this is even more of a reason for being content with a smile and a sense of humor.

Or this from the police officer friend we mentioned earlier:

> A sense of humor in any given stressful situation is always a great attitude to have. I feel that sometimes Bill gets frustrated with his diabetes, and if I can make him laugh a little, he will relax about it. In my job we have to have a sense of humor about the most serious situations, and as my friends and co-workers will tell you, I'm the clown.

The important thing to remember is that the humor should not be directed *at* the diabetic man—especially in the early stages of his disease when he's feeling particularly sensitive and vulnerable. It has to be the two of you laughing *together* about the funny situations that arise in the course of diabetes. Later on, as his mental adjustment to diabetes improves, you'll be surprised to see how his sense of humor grows to the extent that he'll start telling his diabetes "war stories" to friends and laugh with them over some of the strange things he did during an insulin reaction or tell of other diabetically induced comic situations. We still laugh over the time we discovered that a voyeur had been looking through a hole in the wall in an Italian ski resort restroom when June was taking a urine test with TesTape and wonder what he thought was going on. We also remember the time that June—whose language is always the height of decorum—started swearing like a sailor's parrot in our editor's office while in the throes of a blood sugar reaction. Our litany of laughter goes on and on, and so can yours. Humor is always there if you take the time to look for it. And when the diabetic man reaches the happy state in which he can see humor in his condition, it means he has truly accepted it. When he has accepted it, he can control it, and together you can experience many more years of happily humorous events.

Your
DIABETIC SON
· · · ·
Parental Guidance

We don't have to tell you that as a parent of a diabetic son you have your work cut out for you. You know it. Not only do you have to guide your boy through the jungle of childhood and darkest adolescence into successful manhood, but you have to do it with the burden of diabetes on both of your backs. This burden sometimes seems so heavy that it makes every step you take feel as if you're sinking into quicksand. Realizing how heavy the burden is, you may try—especially when your son is young—to take his part of the burden and carry it all yourself. Not only is it impossible for you to do this, but when you try, you keep him from building up the strength he'll need to carry it himself throughout the rest of his life.

Just as in the previous chapter, here we're taking real questions from real people and, as before, collaborating with Dr. Lodewick to provide answers. The difference here is that since children with diabetes are so special and have such unique needs, we've brought in some special people with unique answers—parents of diabetic sons—to share their insider views with you. They are Erica Furman, Gilbert Furman, M.D., and Richard Rubin, Ph.D. Dr. Furman is a pediatrician practicing in Covina, California, and Erica, a former medical technician, is the owner of The Diabetic's Answer, a diabetes supply company also in Covina, California. They are the parents of 8-year-old Joshua, who was diagnosed diabetic at 11 months of age. Dr. Rubin is a Certified Mental Health Counselor and a Certified Diabetes Educator on the staff of the Diabetes Center and Pediatric Diabetes Clinic of Johns Hopkins Hospital in Baltimore, Maryland. His son, Stefan, now 19 years old, has had diabetes for over eleven years.

No one can make your journey through the jungle for you, but these people who've been through it themselves can point out some of the lions and tigers lurking there and show you how to avoid being eaten alive.

—June and Barbara

WHAT YOU'LL FIND HERE

FEELINGS AT TIME OF DIAGNOSIS

DIFFICULTIES OF THERAPY

SOURCES OF HELP

LETTING GO

TEACHING SELF-CARE VIA FAST FOOD

OUTWARD BOUND PROGRAM

MOTIVATION

My son has just been diagnosed diabetic and I'm so confused and upset that I can hardly function. How do I handle it? What do I do? I'm desperate!

June and Barbara: What you're feeling is perfectly normal. The parents of every diabetic child—especially when he's first diagnosed—have felt the same way. Although Gilbert and Erica Furman are both health professionals, when their son became diabetic, they went through an emotional meat grinder identical to the one you're going through now. They've been kind enough to forthrightly share their feelings and experiences with you here, as well as some of the solutions they have worked out. (This was originally written when Joshua was three years old. He is now eight.)

At 11 months, our son Joshua was a happy and sometimes monstrous baby. He loved to play with his two older brothers and often mimicked their vocabulary. He didn't have a care in the world.

As a pediatrician, I was kept busy when the January flu season arrived. One by one, all three of our boys came down with it. Joshua was the last one to become ill. He ran a fever for several days and had an occasional bout of vomiting. He appeared to be taking fluids well, but he continued to get weaker. While my wife, Erica, worried that something was terribly wrong with Joshua, I tried to reassure her that it was just the flu.

That evening, when I checked Joshua for wet diapers, I noticed that he was putting out too much urine for the amount of fluids he was taking in. For the first time, the possibility that my child might have diabetes crossed my mind. (Being a parent and a pediatrician is not always the best combination; there's a tendency to always think the worst.) I could not tell Erica my suspicions. I wanted to be certain before alarming her. So I told her we would watch Joshua overnight and in the morning have him checked out by his pediatrician.

When I entered Joshua's room the next morning, I smelled the unmistakable odor of ketones. He was sicker than ever, and he had the heavy, regular breathing seen with diabetic keto-acidosis (a condition in which ketones appear in the urine). I knew then that there was no other possibility. Joshua had diabetes. And yet, I did not say anything to Erica, perhaps because I was still holding on to a slender hope that my diagnosis could be wrong.

Since I had to make rounds at the hospital that morning, we agreed to meet in my office. When I arrived at the hospital, I called my associate to let him know what was going on. He told me to relax, that my son probably just had the flu; he would check things out. As I made my rounds, I had but one thought— Joshua.

I arrived at the office shortly after Erica and Joshua. His urine sample had already been sent to the lab, so I ran over to check the results. Any hope that I could have been wrong was destroyed: Joshua's urine showed 4 plus sugar and ketones. His blood sugar was 750.

Within minutes, Joshua's pediatrician arrived and took over his treatment. I knew I could no longer handle Joshua's medical care; I was too devastated to make careful, objective medical decisions. Joshua, now comatose, was admitted to the hospital for intravenous fluids and insulin therapy. His treatment was handled by his pediatrician and a pediatric endocrinologist.

When things had settled down and Erica and I were alone with Joshua, I broke the news to her. It was an emotional time for both of us. I felt sad and helpless. Erica was shocked; she couldn't even say the word *diabetes*. But while she felt overwhelmed by the news, in one sense it was a relief; she'd been afraid Joshua had leukemia.

As if we didn't have enough to adjust to, we learned that Joshua's pediatric endocrinologist would be leaving for Austria the next morning to attend a diabetes meeting. Feeling the need to do something and to maintain control, I started becoming involved in Joshua's treatment. I wanted more frequent blood glucose testing than the physician caring for Joshua did. I would order additional tests, and he would cancel them.

By the third day in the hospital, Joshua was off intravenous therapy and responding to treatment. The following day, we met with a diabetes teaching nurse to learn how to use the glucose meter. In her compassionate, down-to-earth way, she made it clear that she understood what we were going through.

By the fifth day, though we still felt anxious about assuming total responsibility for Joshua's care, we decided to take him home. To make things easier, we sent his older brothers, Adam (age eight) and Robbie (age five), to Grandma's house until we had time to settle down into a "normal" routine. The boys were too worried about Joshua to stay away. Erica and I sat down with the boys and explained that Joshua had diabetes. I told them that everyone's body needs insulin to use sugar and that Joshua's body couldn't use sugar without shots because he made no insulin of his own. We explained that there would be certain things that Joshua could not eat. We talked about how everyone would have to help to make things easier. Adam and Robbie felt sad about Joshua, and they were worried about him. They were especially concerned about his need for shots.

Later we learned that Adam and Robbie were afraid that they might get diabetes, too. Even though Adam knew that he couldn't "catch" it, he worried that if he got "really sick like Joshua did" that he could get diabetes. It was some time before the boys became less apprehensive about getting diabetes themselves.

The adjustment period of the first weeks was difficult. We were in constant contact with Joshua's doctor. We went through training sessions with nurses and dietitians; some were helpful, others were terrible. Nothing could adequately prepare us for the realities of trying to control the blood sugar of a one year old. Meals were the biggest problem. Trying to tell Joshua when, what, and how much to eat was impossible. It was also a complete contradiction of everything I had ever told parents about the care of their children. The old adage of "leave the child alone, he will eat if he is hungry" simply would not work in Joshua's case. Attempting to keep Joshua's meals on schedule taxed our creativity, as mealtime became playtime and the kitchen turned into an airport, a garage, or feeding time at the zoo.

Trying to maintain his blood sugar in the normal range would lead to frequent bouts with hypoglycemia (low blood sugar). Letting up on the degree of control would lead to blood sugars in the 400s. It was an exercise in frustration. While we continued to do home blood glucose testing, we found it much easier to focus our attention on the glycosylated hemoglobin (A_1C) test, which reflects the average blood sugars over the past three months. Although Joshua's blood sugar levels were not normal, they did continue to improve from one test period to the next.

Throughout the next year, Joshua continued to make sure that we wouldn't take him, or the diabetes, for granted. One of the more frightening incidents was the night Joshua had a seizure from an insulin reaction. He awoke making the strangest movements, as if he were trying to grab the print pattern off his sheets. His blood sugar was very low—in the 30s. Giving him a glucose gel by mouth and then glucagon by injection, we raised his blood sugar first to 84 and then to 190. His uncontrolled movements continued; he even tried to eat the cardboard box that had contained the glucagon.

It wasn't until 45 minutes later, after we got him to the hospital and administered phenobarbital intravenously, that he calmed down.

For the next week we anxiously awaited the test results while Joshua underwent an extensive neurological evaluation. Fortunately, all of the tests were normal, and Joshua was placed on medication (Tegretol) to try to prevent a recurrence of the hypoglycemic seizures.

Despite an occasional tantrum, Joshua adjusted well to his daily injections. By his second birthday, he had learned to turn on the blood glucose meter himself, push the automatic lancet button, and start the timer on the meter. Rather than fearing syringes and needles, Joshua played with them after getting his shot. Gradually, on his own, he took on more of the tasks of self-management with supervision by his mother and me.

And yet we were frustrated in our attempts to keep Joshua's blood sugar under control. His morning blood glucose level was usually over 300. Attempts to lower it would usually result in a 3 A.M. insulin reaction.

When Joshua was 32 months old, we began to consider using a pump to get better control. After weeks of training, we decided to go ahead. Erica wore a saline-filled pump overnight to see what it was like. She found it tolerable and felt that Joshua would accept it.

The first time I placed the line into his leg, Joshua fought it like a tiger. Gradually, he's done better, but there are still times when putting in the line is a painful experience for both of us.

Today, at age three, Joshua helps with the pump, just as he used to help with his insulin injections. When giving insulin with the pump, we will key in the number of units to be delivered, and Joshua will press "A for acavate" (activate) and do the insulin delivery himself. He will even tell us that he needs insulin.

While the pump has improved his glucose control, it has also increased the need for extremely close monitoring of his blood sugar levels. For us, the improved control is worth the added difficulties. Joshua wants to keep the pump and doesn't want to return to "shots."

Our decision to attempt using the pump was not made lightly. We went through weeks of training and discussion with Joshua's pediatric endocrinologist and his nurse educator. Although the pump has helped us, our experience is not typical.

For very young children, injections are the preferred method of administering insulin.

We are grateful to have three wonderful boys, each with his own special needs. Although Joshua's needs often supersede everything else, we try not to give him special treatment. Things haven't always been that easy for Adam and Robbie. Our plans often revolved around diabetes management. Erica and I had to adjust to a more rigid schedule, keeping an eye on the time to be sure that snacks, testing, and insulin were taken care of. When Joshua would become ill, he needed closer attention than his brothers. Sometimes they were jealous of the special treatment Joshua was getting.

We have tried coping with the situation by being open about the disease and involving the entire family in Joshua's care. Erica has opened a diabetes supply store and teaches parents and family members how to use blood glucose meters. I have become much more involved in the care of young patients with diabetes.

I will usually bring Joshua to the hospital to visit a child or adolescent with newly diagnosed diabetes. The patient then gets a chance to see how well Joshua is coping.

Like many other three year olds, Joshua attends preschool. We've taught his teachers how to recognize signs of hypoglycemia, as well as how to do a blood test and how to administer insulin with the pump. Erica and I are nearby if an emergency should arise, but so far none has.

Living with diabetes—like living with the pump—is a full-time job. There are no vacations. We have found that the cooperation of the entire family makes the job much easier. Joshua is treated as the bright, normal, happy, and loving child he is. He just happens to have diabetes.*

Erica and Gilbert have told us that Joshua is now no longer using the pump. During an active growth period, it stopped being as effective for his blood sugar control. It particularly wasn't covering the nights well. Therefore, about two and a half years ago, they went back to using the needles, with three to four shots a day. It was also true that wearing the pump started to cramp the style and curtail the activities (such as swimming)

---

*Reprinted with permission from *Diabetes Forecast*, July / August 1986. Copyright © 1986 American Diabetes Association, Inc.

of this active, lively boy. His new therapy is working well, and he consistently has good glycohemoglobin tests. This points up the fact that diabetes is not a static condition. It keeps changing, and you must be flexible and change the therapy as needed to keep your son's diabetes in good control and help him have a normal, happy life.

We know if you were able to talk to the Furmans, you'd have many questions to ask. On the following pages we have asked them a few questions synthesized from those we've had from parents of newly diagnosed children. But if there's something important that we haven't covered, Erica—who knows how lost and alone you feel since she's been there herself—invites you to get in touch with her at the Diabetic's Answer, 1126 Grand Avenue, Suite D, Covina, CA 91724 (1-818-915-7773).

What has been the most difficult part of the therapy for Josh to accept? And what has been the hardest for you?

Erica Furman: Josh does very well for the most part. He does get very tired of the testing (who can blame him?), and he sometimes resists when we try to rotate his shot sites. Insulin reactions are difficult. Josh turns into the Incredible Hulk and at times needs several people to hold him down to treat the reaction.

The hardest part of this disease is the daily management. We try very hard to keep Josh a normal child and not let the diabetes rule him or us. At times it is very difficult to differentiate between an insulin reaction and typical childhood tantrum behavior. Although Josh is doing wonderfully for his age, the fear of long-term complications haunts us both. We try to believe that keeping Josh as healthy as possible (relatively normal glycohemoglobins and so on) will allow him to be a candidate when medical science finds that very needed cure.

Where or from whom have you found the most help in dealing with diabetes?

Erica Furman: The support and help we received from the hospital was a joke. I do not recall any diabetes education. I guess they assumed that since Gil and I were in the medical field we knew it all. Our savior was Barbara Cisternino, R.N., from Lifescan (a blood glucose monitor company). Her devotion, love, and caring helped us through the darkest hours. "Grandma Barbara" is now an adopted member of the Furman family.

The next support came from fellow diabetics that I met through the Diabetic's Answer. Talking to them and sharing our mutual concerns was a tremendous help. And yet at times, I still feel alone with Joshua's disease.

Do you have any special advice for mothers and fathers of diabetic boys—especially newly diagnosed diabetic boys?

Erica Furman: The best advice I can give any parents of a diabetic boy is to let go. Don't make your son a cripple because of a manageable disease. Let him take charge—it's his disease. Let him test, give shots, prepare meals, and so on. All of this, of course, should be under strict supervision. Let your son have a normal life. He is a normal boy who just happens to have diabetes!

June and Barbara: Your point about letting your son take charge of his disease is very important—not just for his diabetes but for his whole existence. An article in the *New York Times* by Lawrence Kutner quotes Dr. Arthur L. Kovacs, Dean Emeritus of the California School of Professional Psychology in Los Angeles: "Focusing your life primarily on your children is really doing them a disservice in the long run. They have trouble developing the autonomy that they'll need later in life." You aren't letting go just for the child's benefit, but for your own as well. If a child hasn't developed autonomy, he will try to deprive *you* of *your* freedom, expecting you to always be available for whatever needs he may have. Later he will feel threatened and anxious if you try to reclaim your own autonomous existence and pursue your own interests in life, such as moving to a new area or remarrying upon divorce or death of your spouse.

The article points out that you must start preparing your children for independence at an early age. Dr. Florence Kaslow, the director of the Florida Couples and Family Institute in West Palm Beach, suggests that you "encourage your children to do activities away from, as well as with, the family at an early age. Do things without your children, including spending weekends away, while they're still young."

You should also be on the lookout for early signs—often very subtle ones—of inappropriate dependency. As Dr. Rita P. Underberg, a clinical psychologist and clinical professor of psychiatry at the University of Rochester, states: "You expect young teenagers to say, 'Don't tell me what to do.' If your teenager keeps asking you to make his or her routine choices, that may be an indicator of future problems separating."

Admittedly, the problem with teenage boys is far more likely to be one of rebellion than of overdependency. Just recently we heard the story of a boy who delighted in terrorizing his mother by shooting up a lot of insulin and eating a hot fudge sundae in front of her. Food is often a major battleground for diabetic teenagers and their parents. For tactical information on this subject, we've called in an expert (both professionally and personally)—Dr. Richard Rubin.

My son, who's had diabetes for six years, is now a teenager and wants to go to fast food places with his friends. My problem is that I know he's going to run his blood sugar up trying to "fit in." What can I do?

Dr. Richard Rubin: I share this problem with every parent who has a child with diabetes over the age of 10. Isn't it our duty to keep our children from eating food that's not good for them? That's what we tried to do when our children were younger. Why should we stop now? The reason we have to stop, or at least adjust our approach, is simple: our kids are growing up and are—for better or worse—no longer completely under our wing. To put it bluntly, the question isn't whether our kids are going to eat junk food—they are. The question is, how are we going to deal with it?

It's a time of change, for us and for them. And for all of us, the focus shifts to preparing for self-care. At this age we will have a say in how our kids live with their diabetes for another six to eight years. Then, for the next 60 years or so, what they do will be completely up to them. If we try to maintain complete control over what they do now, we do them a great disservice. We deprive them of the opportunity to learn about self-care, gradually and gently, while we are still there to help.

To prepare our children for a healthy future, we have to help them learn to make decisions now. This isn't easy, but it is essential. Their choices will not always be the ones we would make. Any new skill is really difficult to master. Remember when your son was first learning to ride a two-wheeler? He needed you right there with him, running along beside him as he weaved along and took his inevitable tumbles. You couldn't ride the bike for him, but you had to be there to help. Helping our children learn to balance their lives with diabetes is infinitely harder than helping them learn to ride a bike, but the principles are the same. We must let our kids test themselves, make mistakes, and learn from their mistakes. The experience of years of working with adults who had diabetes as children convinces me that any other approach guarantees disaster. I've seen too many adults who aren't able to manage their lives with diabetes because they never had the chance to practice when they were children. Their diabetes was their parents' responsibility, and they missed that critical period for developing the capacity to take care of themselves.

So what can we do to help our preteen and early teenage children learn to live with the fast food frenzies? Here are a few practical tips I've learned over the years through a combination of personal and clinical experience.

- Keep your goal in mind. It's to start your son on the path to good self-care, not to keep him from eating things he shouldn't eat. Let him satisfy some of his junk food cravings.

- Find out some of his food cravings. Help him learn to balance this need with his need for fairly normal blood sugars. The key is to have a list of "adjust and do's," not "do's and don'ts."

- Play "let's make a deal." He can have dinner at a restaurant with his friends after the matinee as a trade-off for any one of a list of choices (for instance, you meet him at the restaurant for a check-in, he tests blood sugar before eating and adjusts his insulin dosage accordingly, etc.).

Remember, the issue isn't morality; it's reality. There are no rights or wrongs, only results. If you can help your son develop a system that gives him occasional junk food treats and keeps his blood sugars on a fairly even keel, you have given him a wonderful gift—a process for living well with diabetes.

June and Barbara: Another wonderful gift Richard Rubin's son has received is the gift of increased self-confidence and self-knowledge that comes from having participated in an Outward Bound program under the auspices of Dr. Raymonde Dumont-Herskowitz of the Joslin Diabetes Center. These sessions of 5 to 120 days take place at the Hurricane Island Outward Bound School on the coast of Maine. The activities include sailing expeditions, a high ropes course, rock climbing, and daily running or swimming. As reported in a study in *Diabetic Medicine*, so far six courses have been taught to a total of 56 students with Type I diabetes. Based on psychological profiles and personal correspondence from the participants, they almost universally felt it was a positive experience that "expanded their knowledge of self-care and increased their determination to meet the ongoing challenges of diabetes." Not only did they gain self-confidence and self-esteem, but they learned that diabetes need not stand in your way of doing the things you want to do. The following case studies of participants present convincing evidence of the benefits of the Outward Bound experience.

Case 1

A 17-year-old young woman with longstanding brittle diabetes and a history of recurrent diabetic ketoacidosis agreed to participate in the program. During the course a minor viral illness led to hyperglycemia with large ketonuria. With intensive additional insulin injection of up to 20 U every 3 hours, and continuous sips of fluids, she was able to avert diabetic ketoacidosis and dehydration. This was her first experience with successful self-management when ill. Since completion of her course, she has had sustained improvement of her blood glucose control, with a glycosylated hemoglobin improving from around 20.0 down to 14%.

Case 2

A 14-year-old girl with monthly recurrent diabetic ketoacidosis had recently been placed in foster care due to a turbulent family situation. Struggling on the high ropes course, she was heard to brace herself with "I've lived through a difficult year, I can deal with this too!" Upon returning home, she has continued to utilize this (now conscious) awareness of her strengths, to work through her troubled home life, and since then she has not been hospitalized for ketoacidosis.

Case 3

A 19-year-old young man had shown a haphazard approach to diabetes care, with little monitoring, no insulin dose adjustments, and no meal plan. Throughout the course, the group was faced with his constant need to occupy center stage. Humorous and friendly strategies were developed for containing him, while his skills and contributions to team efforts were overtly appreciated. A group discussion led him to tell us that his behavior stemmed from a deep wish to capture the attention of an alcoholic father. Having previously denied any problems, he now related trouble with the law, drinking, and frequent use of various noninjectable "street drugs." Other group members, in an emotionally charged experience, gave him understanding and support. Two other participants cried with him about their own fathers' alcoholism. Six months later, he continues to care for his health, to do well in college, and has taken no drugs or excess alcohol.

If you have an adolescent son you think would benefit from the Outward Bound experience, you can write for information to Dr. Dumont-Herskowitz, Joslin Diabetes Center, One Joslin Place, Boston, MA 02215.

Just as for an adult, motivation is vital for young people who need to make changes to improve their diabetes control.

How can I motivate my teenage son to take better care of his diabetes?

Dr. Lodewick: Let's first talk about motivation in general. Motivation usually comes when a person finds a purpose in his life, something that gives his life meaning. Motivation is difficult for some to achieve, but for others it's almost a way of life. I can cite the example of a man who met defeat after defeat in his business, in a run for Legislature, in an emotional breakdown, in a run for the Senate, and in a run for the Vice-Presidency. Finally, he became President of the United States. His name is Abraham Lincoln. Despite all his failures, he never gave up. He felt in his heart that he could have a positive effect on the history of his country. Motivation par excellence!

Now back to the practical world of diabetes. How do you motivate your son? I don't know for sure. It has to come from within himself. Concentrate on his desire for pleasure: let him know that by caring for himself, he will feel better and get more enjoyment from life. Work on his desire for autonomy: let him know you will stop nagging him when he starts caring for himself. And work on his desire for achievement, possibly rewarding him for achieving good blood sugar levels or glycohemoglobin tests.

Try to get him to define what he wants out of his life. What kind of work would he like to do? Having a well-defined future will help him want to take good care of himself so he can be around to experience it. He'll want to prevent the complications that can take place, keep himself in shape for a good job and a good marriage. Don't badger him, just try to get him to focus on his goals. Don't harp on him for failing to get perfect control of blood sugars. As Abe Lincoln failed, so do all human beings. With diabetes it's even tougher, since we don't have methods of achieving perfect control. Allow him some failure. A certain amount of failure is inevitable, and acknowledging this fact will take the stress off him, especially when growth, physical maturity, and his search for self-identification are all hitting him at once. More important, be sympathetic, supportive, and understanding. In time, he will pull through—and so will you!

POSTSCRIPT

It's a Wise Child

It was Christmas morning and—as was the family tradition—Richard Rubin was making three wishes for his family for the following year. The first two were for smaller things such as finding the right computer and having the whole family learn how to use it easily. He saved the big one for last. He said to his son, "I wish you didn't have diabetes."

"I'll go along with the first two wishes," said his son. "But not the third one."

Dr. Rubin's jaw fell. "What are you talking about?"

"I'm not sure I can put it in words. I don't like having diabetes; I hate it. But somehow it has forced me to learn how to take care of myself. I wouldn't give up knowing how to do that for anything in the world."

May your son gain that knowledge—and the wisdom to realize its priceless value.

AFTERWORD

· · · ·

Profile Encourage

It was said simply in the New Testament, "Physician, heal thyself." It was said more wordily by Cicero: "Do not imitate those unskillful physicians who profess to possess the healing art in the diseases of others, but are unable to cure themselves." And it was said pungently in *The Neurotic's Notebook*: "Most psychiatrists are such poor advertisements for themselves—like dermatologists with acne."

Throughout this book you've been given a lot of advice on how to live your life as a diabetic man. Digesting, understanding, and following all this advice will take a certain amount of effort on your part. How do you know that effort will be worthwhile? What if you extend yourself to do everything exactly the way you're supposed to and it just doesn't work? What if several years down the road you wind up unhealthy and with diabetic complications, despite all you've done to avoid it?

Although there are no guarantees in life, there are some fairly sure things that have great odds in your favor. The fact that the advice in this book works is one of them. We know because we have an example of someone who has been following this advice for 23 years, and as a result he is the living, breathing, and running-around proof that it does work—Peter A. Lodewick, M.D. He is one physician who has truly healed himself.

Read this encouraging physical profile and smile, secure in the knowledge that you can have one just as good if you put your mind, body, and spirit to it.

Dr. Lodewick's Physical Profile

Age: 49 years
Age at diabetes onset: 26 years
Year diagnosed: 1968
Duration: 23 years

Health Status

	Normal Range
Blood pressure: 138/82 mmHg	Under 140/90
Electrocardiogram: Normal	—
Total cholesterol: 189 mgm%	Less than 200
HDL cholesterol: 61 mgm%	Over 40
LDL cholesterol: 117 mgm%	Under 130
Triglycerides: 44 mgm%	Under 150
Average fasting blood sugar: 140 mg%	Under 100
Glycohemoglobin: 8.5%	4.4 to 8.2
Urine protein: negative	Negative

Family history: Negative for diabetes in large family.

Exercise: Jogging 3–5 days per week, 14–20 miles per week, 750–820 miles per year.
Tennis: Outplays high school tennis players.

Diet: 2000–2400 calories per day. Low in fat.

Physical exams: One per year.

Eye exams: One per year. No retinopathy present.

Stress electrocardiograms: Every five years. No heart disease present.

Dr. Lodewick: I appreciate your kind remarks about the state of my health. I must admit, though, that I've been fortunate. There are still many things we don't know about diabetes, and there are people out there who do get complications or don't get adequate control despite their greatest efforts. That's why we still need to find answers so we can get better treatment methods and ultimately find the causes of diabetes so the ultimate cure—prevention—will be ours!

References and Suggested Readings

Anderson, James. *Diabetes: A Practical New Guide to Healthy Living.* New York: Warner Books, 1981.

Atkins, Robert C. *Dr. Atkins' Diet Revolution: The High Calorie Way to Stay Thin Forever.* New York: McKay, 1972.

Bailey, Covert. *Fit or Fat Target Diet.* Boston: Houghton Mifflin, 1984.

Biermann, June, and Toohey, Barbara. *Diabetic's Book: All Your Questions Answered.* Revised Edition. Los Angeles: Jeremy P. Tarcher, 1990.

Biermann, June, and Toohey, Barbara. *Diabetic's Sports and Exercise Book.* New York: Lippincott, 1977.

Biermann, June, and Toohey, Barbara. *Diabetic's Total Health Book.* Revised Edition. Los Angeles: Jeremy P. Tarcher, 1988.

Biermann, June, and Toohey, Barabara. *The Peripatetic Diabetic.* Revised Edition. Los Angeles: Jeremy P. Tarcher, 1983.

Castine, Jacqueline. *Recovery from Rescuing.* Deerfield Beach, Florida: Health Communications, 1989.

Cooper, Kenneth N. *Running Without Fear: How to Reduce the Risk of Heart Attack and Sudden Death During Aerobic Exercise.* New York: M. Evans, 1985.

Ehret, Charles F., and Scanlon, Lynne. *Overcoming Jet Lag.* New York: Berkley Books, 1983.

Ellis, Albert. *How to Stubbornly Refuse to Make Yourself Miserable Over Anything—Yes, Anything!* New York: Lyle Stuart, 1988.

Ferguson, James M. *Habits Not Diets.* Palo Alto, California: Bull Publishing Company, 1988.

Glasser, William. *Positive Addiction.* New York: Harper & Row, 1985.

Hendler, Sheldon. *Complete Guide to Anti-Aging Nutrients.* New York: Simon & Schuster, 1985.

Jovanovic, Lois, Biermann, June, and Toohey, Barbara. *The Diabetic Woman.* Los Angeles: Jeremy P. Tarcher, 1987.

Lodewick, Peter. *A Doctor Looks at Diabetes: His and Yours.* Revised Edition. Waltham, Massachusetts: R.M.I. Corporation, 1988.

Mirkin, Gabe, and Shangold, Mona M. *The Complete Sportsmedicine Book.* Boston: Little, Brown & Company, 1978.

Pelletier, Kenneth R. *Mind as Healer, Mind as Slayer: A Holistic Approach to Preventing Stress Disorders.* New York: Delacorte, 1977.

Pritikin, Nathan. *Diet for Runners.* New York: Simon & Schuster, 1985.

Pritikin, Nathan, with McGrady, Patrick M. *Pritikin Program for Diet and Exercise.* New York: Bantam Books, 1980.

Reinisch, June, and Beasley, June. *The Kinsey Institute New Report on Sex.* New York: St. Martin's, 1990.

Schaef, Anne Wilson. *When Society Becomes an Addict.* San Francisco: Harper & Row, 1987.

Sheehan, George. *Running and Being: The Total Experience.* New York: Simon & Schuster, 1978.

Shekerjian, Denise. *Uncommon Genius: How Great Ideas Are Born.* New York: Viking Press, 1990.

Appendix A

CONVERSION CHART of mg/dL to mmol/L

mg/dL	mmol/L
720	40
540	30
360	20
270	15
216	12
198	11
180	10
162	9
144	8
126	7
108	6
90	5
72	4
54	3
36	2

Appendix B

DIFFERENCES BETWEEN INSULIN-DEPENDENT (TYPE I) AND NON-INSULIN-DEPENDENT (TYPE II) DIABETES

	Insulin-Dependent	Non-Insulin-Dependent
Age of onset	Usually less than 20 years, but can be any age	Usually over 30 years, but a small number of cases develop the disease before the age of 30
"Tip-off"	Abrupt onset of symptoms with weight loss	Slow onset of symptoms, sometimes with weight gain
Family history	At first, may be none, but as years pass, family history may manifest itself as a factor	Commonly a factor
Stability	Not very stable; must closely monitor changes in insulin, exercise, and food intake, which affect blood sugar markedly	More stable; changes in insulin, exercise, and food have much less dramatic effect on blood sugar
Control of disease	Difficult	Less difficult
Complications	May occur	May occur
Diet	Vitally important	Important and may determine whether or not patient needs insulin or pills
Insulin need	Yes—100%	Needed in only 20–30% of cases
Need for pills	No	Sometimes

Appendix C

AMERICAN DIABETES ASSOCIATION AFFILIATES

ALABAMA

AMERICAN DIABETES
ASSOCIATION
ALABAMA AFFILIATE, INC.
3 Office Park Circle, Suite 115
Birmingham, AL 35223
(205) 870-5172 or (205) 870-5173
800-824-7891 (Toll Free)

ALASKA

AMERICAN DIABETES
ASSOCIATION
ALASKA AFFILIATE, INC.
201 E. 3rd Avenue, Suite 301
Anchorage, AK 99501
(907) 276-3607

ARIZONA

AMERICAN DIABETES
ASSOCIATION
ARIZONA AFFILIATE, INC.
7337 North 19th Avenue,
Room 404
Phoenix, AZ 85021
(602) 995-1515

ARKANSAS

AMERICAN DIABETES
ASSOCIATION
ARKANSAS AFFILIATE, INC.
11500 N. Rodney Paraham
Executive Suite Bldg.,
Suites 19 & 20
Little Rock, AR 72212
(501) 221-7444

CALIFORNIA

AMERICAN DIABETES
ASSOCIATION
CALIFORNIA AFFILIATE, INC.
2031 Howe Avenue, Suite 250
Sacramento, CA 95825
(916) 925-0199

COLORADO

AMERICAN DIABETES
ASSOCIATION
COLORADO AFFILIATE, INC.
2450 S. Downing Street
Denver, CO 80210
(303) 778-7556

CONNECTICUT

AMERICAN DIABETES
ASSOCIATION
CONNECTICUT AFFILIATE, INC.
40 South Street
West Hartford, CT 06110
(203) 249-4232 or
1-800-842-6323

DELAWARE

AMERICAN DIABETES
ASSOCIATION
DELAWARE AFFILIATE, INC.
2713 Lancaster Avenue
Wilmington, DE 19805
(302) 656-0030

DISTRICT OF COLUMBIA

AMERICAN DIABETES
ASSOCIATION
WASHINGTON, D.C. AREA
AFFILIATE, INC.
1819 H Street, N.W., Suite 1200
Washington, D.C. 20006-3603
(202) 331-8303

FLORIDA

AMERICAN DIABETES
ASSOCIATION
FLORIDA AFFILIATE, INC.
P.O. Box 915559 (mailing address)
2180 W. State Route 434,
Suite 2100 (street address)
Longwood, FL 32791-5559
(407) 862-1965 or
1-800-432-5698

GEORGIA

AMERICAN DIABETES
ASSOCIATION
GEORGIA AFFILIATE, INC.
3783 Presidential Parkway,
Suite 102
Atlanta, GA 30340
(404) 454-8401

HAWAII

AMERICAN DIABETES
ASSOCIATION
HAWAII AFFILIATE, INC.
510 South Beretania Street
Honolulu, HI 96813
(808) 521-5677

IDAHO

AMERICAN DIABETES
ASSOCIATION
IDAHO AFFILIATE, INC.
1528 Vista
Boise, ID 83705
(208) 342-2774

ILLINOIS

AMERICAN DIABETES
ASSOCIATION
DOWNSTATE ILLINOIS
AFFILIATE, INC.
965 N. Water Street
Decatur, IL 62523
(217) 422-8228

AMERICAN DIABETES
ASSOCIATION
NORTHERN ILLINOIS
AFFILIATE, INC.
6 N. Michigan Avenue, Suite 1202
Chicago, IL 60602
(312) 346-1805

INDIANA

AMERICAN DIABETES
ASSOCIATION
INDIANA AFFILIATE, INC.
222 S. Downey Avenue, Suite 320
Indianapolis, IN 46219
(317) 352-9226

IOWA

AMERICAN DIABETES
ASSOCIATION
IOWA AFFILIATE, INC.
3829 71st Street, Suite A
Des Moines, IA 50322
(515) 276-2237 or
1-800-678-4232

KANSAS

AMERICAN DIABETES
ASSOCIATION
KANSAS AFFILIATE, INC.
3210 E. Douglas
Wichita, KS 67208
(316) 684-6091

KENTUCKY

AMERICAN DIABETES
ASSOCIATION
KENTUCKY AFFILIATE, INC.
745 West Main, Suite 150
Louisville, KY 40202
(502) 589-3837

LOUISIANA

AMERICAN DIABETES
ASSOCIATION
LOUISIANA AFFILIATE, INC.
9420 Lindale Avenue, Suite B
Baton Rouge, LA 70815
(504) 927-7732

MAINE

AMERICAN DIABETES
ASSOCIATION
MAINE AFFILIATE, INC.
P.O. Box 2208 (mailing address)
c/o S. Parish Congregational
Church (street address)
9 Church Street
Augusta, ME 04330-2208
(207) 623-2232

MARYLAND

AMERICAN DIABETES
ASSOCIATION
MARYLAND AFFILIATE, INC.
3701 Old Court Road, Suite 19
Baltimore, MD 21208
(301) 486-5516

MASSACHUSETTS

AMERICAN DIABETES
ASSOCIATION
MASSACHUSETTS AFFILIATE,
INC.
190 N. Main Street
Natick, MA 01760
(508) 655-6900

MICHIGAN

AMERICAN DIABETES
ASSOCIATION
MICHIGAN AFFILIATE, INC.
The Clausen Building North Unit
23100 Providence Drive,
Suite 400
Southfield, MI 48075
(313) 552-0480

MINNESOTA

AMERICAN DIABETES
ASSOCIATION
MINNESOTA AFFILIATE, INC.
715 Florida Avenue South
715 Florida West Building
Golden Valley, MN 55426
(612) 920-6796

MISSISSIPPI

AMERICAN DIABETES
ASSOCIATION
MISSISSIPPI AFFILIATE, INC.
16 Northtown Drive, Suite 100
Jackson, MS 39211
(601) 957-7878

MISSOURI

AMERICAN DIABETES
ASSOCIATION
MISSOURI AFFILIATE, INC.
P.O. Box 1674 (mailing address)
213 Adams Street
Jefferson City, MO 65102
(314) 636-5552

MONTANA

AMERICAN DIABETES
ASSOCIATION
MONTANA AFFILIATE, INC.
Box 2411 (mailing address)
Great Falls, MT 59403
600 Central Plaza,
Suite 304 (street address)
Great Falls, MT 59401
(406) 761-0908

NEBRASKA

AMERICAN DIABETES
ASSOCIATION
NEBRASKA AFFILIATE, INC.
2730 S. 114th Street
Omaha, NE 68144
(402) 333-5556

NEVADA

AMERICAN DIABETES
ASSOCIATION
NEVADA AFFILIATE, INC.
4045 S. Spencer, Suite A-62
Las Vegas, NV 89119
(702) 369-9995

NEW HAMPSHIRE

AMERICAN DIABETES
ASSOCIATION
NEW HAMPSHIRE
AFFILIATE, INC.
P.O. Box 595
(mailing address)
Manchester, NH 03105
104 Middle Street (street address)
Manchester, NH 03101
(603) 627-9579

NEW JERSEY

AMERICAN DIABETES
ASSOCIATION
NEW JERSEY AFFILIATE, INC.
P.O. Box 6423 (mailing address)
312 N. Adamsville Road
(street address)
Bridgewater, NJ 08807
(201) 725-7878

NEW MEXICO

AMERICAN DIABETES
ASSOCIATION
NEW MEXICO AFFILIATE, INC.
525 San Pedro, N.E., Suite 108
Albuquerque, NM 87108
(505) 266-5716

NEW YORK

AMERICAN DIABETES
ASSOCIATION
NEW YORK DOWNSTATE
AFFILIATE, INC.
505 8th Avenue
New York, NY 10018
(212) 947-9707

NEW YORK (cont'd)

AMERICAN DIABETES
ASSOCIATION
NEW YORK UPSTATE
AFFILIATE, INC.
P.O. Box 1037 (mailing address)
Syracuse, NY 13201
115 E. Jefferson Street
(street address)
Syracuse, NY 13202
(315) 472-9111

NORTH CAROLINA

AMERICAN DIABETES
ASSOCIATION
NORTH CAROLINA
AFFILIATE, INC.
2315-A Sunset Avenue
Rocky Mount, NC 27801
(919) 937-4121

NORTH DAKOTA

AMERICAN DIABETES
ASSOCIATION
NORTH DAKOTA
AFFILIATE, INC.
P.O. Box 234 (mailing address)
Grand Forks, ND 58206-0234
101 N. 3rd Street, Suite 502
(street address)
Grand Forks, ND 58201
(701) 746-4427

OHIO

AMERICAN DIABETES
ASSOCIATION
OHIO AFFILIATE, INC.
705L Lakeview Plaza Court
Columbus, OH 43085
(614) 436-1917

OKLAHOMA

AMERICAN DIABETES
ASSOCIATION
OKLAHOMA AFFILIATE, INC.
Warren Professional Building
6465 S. Yale Avenue, Suite 423
Tulsa, OK 74136
(918) 492-3839 or
1-800-722-5448

OREGON

AMERICAN DIABETES
ASSOCIATION
OREGON AFFILIATE, INC.
3607 S.W. Corbett Street
Portland, OR 97201
(503) 228-0849

PENNSYLVANIA

AMERICAN DIABETES
ASSOCIATION
GREATER PHILADELPHIA
AFFILIATE, INC.
21 South Fifth Street
The Bourse, Suite 570
Philadelphia, PA 19106
(215) 627-7718

AMERICAN DIABETES
ASSOCIATION
MID-PENNSYLVANIA
AFFILIATE, INC.
2045 Westgate Drive, Suite 106
Bethlehem, PA 18017
(215) 867-6660

AMERICAN DIABETES
ASSOCIATION
WESTERN PENNSYLVANIA
AFFILIATE, INC.
4617 Winthrop Street
Pittsburgh, PA 15213
(412) 682-3392

PUERTO RICO

AMERICAN DIABETES
ASSOCIATION
PUERTO RICO AFFILIATE, INC.
Avenue Jesus T. Pineiro
(Central) 1161 Altos
Puerto Nuevo, Puerto Rico 00920
(809) 793-1276

RHODE ISLAND

AMERICAN DIABETES
ASSOCIATION
RHODE ISLAND AFFILIATE, INC.
Warwick Executive Park
250 Centerville Road
Warwick, RI 02886
(401) 738-5570

SOUTH CAROLINA

AMERICAN DIABETES
ASSOCIATION
SOUTH CAROLINA
AFFILIATE, INC.
P.O. Box 50782 (mailing address)
2838 Devine Street
Columbia, SC 29250
(803) 799-4246

SOUTH DAKOTA

AMERICAN DIABETES
ASSOCIATION
SOUTH DAKOTA AFFILIATE, INC.
P.O. Box 659 (mailing address)
Sioux Falls, SD 57101
1524 W. 20th Street
(street address)
Sioux Falls, SD 57105
(605) 335-7670

TENNESSEE

AMERICAN DIABETES
ASSOCIATION
TENNESSEE AFFILIATE, INC.
Green Hills Court
4004 Hillsboro Road, Suite B-216
Nashville, TN 37215
(615) 298-9919

TEXAS

AMERICAN DIABETES
ASSOCIATION
TEXAS AFFILIATE, INC.
8140 N. Mopac, Bldg. 1, Suite 130
Austin, TX 78759
(512) 343-6981

UTAH

AMERICAN DIABETES
ASSOCIATION
UTAH AFFILIATE, INC.
643 East 400 South
Salt Lake City, UT 84102
(801) 363-3024

VERMONT

AMERICAN DIABETES
ASSOCIATION
VERMONT AFFILIATE, INC.
431 Pine Street
Maltex Building
Burlington, VT 05401
(802) 862-3882

VIRGINIA

AMERICAN DIABETES
ASSOCIATION
VIRGINIA AFFILIATE, INC.
404 8th Street, N.E., Suite C
Charlottesville, VA 22901
(804) 293-4953

WASHINGTON

AMERICAN DIABETES
ASSOCIATION
WASHINGTON AFFILIATE, INC.
3201 Fremont Avenue North
Seattle, WA 98103
(206) 632-4576 or
1-800-628-8808

WEST VIRGINIA

AMERICAN DIABETES
ASSOCIATION
WEST VIRGINIA AFFILIATE, INC.
P.O. Box 4512
Charleston, WV 25364
(304) 925-0161 or
1-800-642-3055

WISCONSIN

AMERICAN DIABETES
ASSOCIATION
WISCONSIN AFFILIATE, INC.
10721 W. Capitol Drive
Milwaukee, WI 53222
(414) 464-9395

WYOMING

AMERICAN DIABETES
ASSOCIATION
WYOMING AFFILIATE, INC.
2526 6th Avenue North
Billings, MT 59101
(307) 638-3578 or (307) 237-2325

Appendix D

CANADIAN DIABETES ASSOCIATION DIVISIONS

National Office, 78 Bond Street, Toronto, Ontario, M5B 2J8

Divisions

ALBERTA

10240 124th Street, Room 305
Edmonton, Alberta T5N 3W6
(403) 482-2307

BRITISH COLUMBIA

1091 West 8th Avenue
Vancouver, B.C. V6H 2V3
(604) 732-1331

MANITOBA

283 Portage Avenue, 2nd Floor
Winnipeg, Manitoba R3B 2B5
(204) 943-7529

NEW BRUNSWICK

259 Brunswick Street
Fredericton, New Brunswick
E3B 1G8
(506) 454-7118

NEWFOUNDLAND

103 Le Marchant Road
P.O. Box 9130
St. John's, Newfoundland
A1A 2X3
(709) 754-0953

NOVA SCOTIA

1221 Barrington Street
Halifax, Nova Scotia B3J 1Y2
(902) 421-1444

ONTARIO

747 Baseline Road East
London, Ontario N6C 2R6
(519) 668-2782

PRINCE EDWARD ISLAND

Box 133
Charlottetown, Prince Edward
Island C1A 7K2
(902) 894-3005

QUEBEC

180, boul. René-Lévesque Est,
Suite 200
Montréal, Quebec H2X 1N6
(514) 398-0955

SASKATCHEWAN

104-2301 Avenue C.N.
Saskatoon, Saskatchewan
S7L 5Z5
(306) 933-1238

Appendix E

Directions for Using the Glucagon Emergency Kit

Glucagon

Glucagon is a prescription drug used in emergencies to increase blood glucose levels in severe insulin reactions (low blood glucose). Low blood glucose can result in convulsions.

Glucagon allows the body to use stored sugar (glycogen) in the liver for energy.

Here are some important facts to remember:

Glucagon is used only for treating severe insulin reactions (low blood glucose) in people with diabetes mellitus who are unable to swallow.

Glucagon is injected in the same way as insulin.

Glucagon may cause nausea and vomiting after administration.

Glucagon is supplied in powder form with accompanying syringe containing diluting solution. This is called a Glucagon Emergency Kit.

Do not use a bottle of glucagon after the date given on the label of the bottle.

Become familiar with instructions for using the Glucagon Emergency Kit before an emergency happens.

Directions for Using the Glucagon Emergency Kit

1. Remove the flip-off seal from the vial (bottle) of glucagon. Wipe the rubber stopper with alcohol swab.

2. Remove the needle protector from the syringe, and inject entire contents of the syringe into vial of glucagon.

3. Remove syringe and shake vial gently until solution is clear.

4. Using the same syringe, withdraw entire solution from the vial.

TO ADMINISTER GLUCAGON

5. Select an injection site: the abdomen, buttocks, upper and outer thigh, or the fatty part of the back of the upper arm.

6. Wipe site with alcohol pad.

7. Pinch up the area of skin and inject the needle at a 90° angle.

8. Inject the entire dose of glucagon. (Note: if recommended by a doctor, inject only one half the dose if the person is a small child.)

OTHER INSTRUCTIONS

Turn the person who received the injection on one side in case vomiting should occur. Do not leave the person alone.

If the person does not wake after 15 to 20 minutes, repeat the injection, and call a doctor as soon as possible.

If the person wakes up and is able to swallow, give a fast-acting carbohydrate (such as regular soft drinks or orange juice) and a long-acting carbohydrate (such as crackers and cheese or meat sandwich).

Reprinted with permission of Eli Lilly and Company from *Managing Your Diabetes—Advisory 2.*

Appendix F

AMSLER GRID

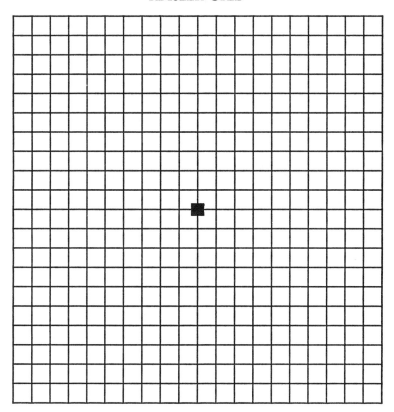

Directions:

1. Use with reading glasses at reading distance.

2. Cover one eye.

3. Look at center dot.

4. Note irregularities (wavy, size, gray, fuzzy).

5. Test other eye.

IF IRREGULARITIES OCCUR, CALL YOUR DOCTOR'S OFFICE IMMEDIATELY.

Appendix G

GLYCEMIC INDEX

The Glycemic Index is basically a classification of how high and how fast the blood sugar is raised by individual carbohydrate foods. The index compares the way carbohydrate foods raise blood sugar with the way straight glucose raises it. Glucose, the form of sugar in the blood, is assigned an index number of 100.

Generally speaking, for a diabetic a low (slow-releasing) Glycemic Index food is preferred to a high (fast-releasing) Glycemic Index food. The chart on the following pages shows the Glycemic Index of some foods that have been tested.

Simple Sugars

Fructose—20
Sucrose—59

Honey—87
Glucose—100

Fruits

Apples—39
Oranges—40
Orange juice—48

Bananas—62
Raisins—64

Starchy Vegetables

Sweet potatoes—48
Yams—51
Beets—64
White potatoes—70

Instant potatoes—80
Carrots—92
Parsnips—97

Dairy Products

Skim milk—32
Whole milk—34

Ice cream—36
Yogurt—36

Legumes

Soybeans—15
Lentils—29
Kidney beans—29
Black-eyed peas—33

Garbanzos—36
Lima beans—36
Baked beans—40
Frozen peas—51

Pasta, Corn, Rice, Bread

Whole-wheat pasta—42
White pasta—50
Sweet corn—59
Brown rice—66

White bread—69
Whole-wheat bread—72
White rice—72

Breakfast Cereals

Oatmeal—49
All-Bran—51
Swiss Muesli—66

Shredded wheat—67
Cornflakes—80

Miscellaneous

Peanuts—13
Sausages—28
Fish sticks—38
Tomato soup—38

Sponge cake—46
Potato chips—51
Mars bars—68

Appendix H

DRUGS THAT CAUSE SEXUAL DYSFUNCTION

Drug	Adverse Effect
Alcohol abuse	Impotence; decreased desire; orgasmic problems
Alprazolam (Xanax)	Inhibition of orgasm; delayed or no ejaculation
Amitriptyline (Elavil and others)	Loss of desire; impotence; no ejaculation
Amoxapine (Asendin)	Loss of desire; impotence; retrograde, painful or no ejaculation
Amphetamines (Tenuate, Plegine, Fastin, and others)	Chronic abuse: impotence; delayed or no ejaculation in men and no orgasm in women
Anticholinergics (Bentyl, Ditropan, Mesopin, and others)	Impotence
Antihistamines	Decreased desire; impotence
Atenolol (Tenormin)	Impotence
Baclofen (Lioresal)	Impotence
Barbiturates	Decreased desire; impotence
Beta-blockers (Tenormin, Inderol, Corgard, Lopressor, and others)	Impotence
Carbamazepine (Tegretol)	Impotence
Chlorodiazepoxide (Librium)	Decreased desire
Chlorpromazine (Thorazine and others)	Decreased desire; impotence; no ejaculation; priapism
Chlorthalidone (Hygroton)	Decreased desire; impotence

Drug	Adverse Effect
Cimetidine (Tagamet)	Decreased desire; impotence
Clofibrate (Atromid-S)	Decreased desire; impotence
Clonidine (Catapres)	Impotence; inhibition of orgasm (women)
Cocaine abuse	Loss of desire; inhibition of orgasm with high doses
Danazol (Danocrin)	Increased or decreased desire
Decongestants	Erectile dysfunction
Desipramine (Norpramin, Pertofrane)	Decreased desire; impotence; difficult ejaculation and painful orgasm
Diazepam (Valium)	Decreased desire; delayed ejaculation
Digoxin (Lanoxin)	Decreased desire; impotence
Diphenhydramine (Benadryl)	Impotence; decreased desire
Disopyramide (Norpace)	Impotence
Disulfiram (Antabuse)	Decreased desire; impotence
Doxepin (Sinequan, Adapin)	Decreased desire; ejaculatory dysfunction
Estrogens (Premarin, Ogen)	Decreased desire in men
Guanabenz (Wytensin)	Impotence
Guanadrel (Hylorel)	Decreased desire; delayed or retrograde ejaculation; impotence
Guanethidine (Ismelin)	Impotence; no ejaculation
Haloperidol (Haldol)	Impotence; painful ejaculation
Heroin abuse	Decreased desire; impotence; retarded ejaculation; delayed orgasm
Hydralazine (Apresoline and others)	Impotence; priapism
Hydroxyprogesterone caproate (Delalutin)	Impotence
Imipramine (Tofranil and others)	Decreased desire; impotence; painful ejaculation; delayed orgasm in women
Levodopa (Dopar and others)	No ejaculation

Drug	Adverse Effect
Lithium (Eskalith and others)	Decreased desire; impotence
Marijuana	Decreased desire; impotence
Mesoridazine (Serentil)	No ejaculation
Methadone	Erectile problems
Methyldopa (Aldomet)	Decreased desire; impotence; delayed or no ejaculation or orgasm
Metoclopramide (Reglan)	Erectile problems
Metoprolol (Lopressor)	Decreased desire; impotence
Metronidozole (Flagyl)	Erectile problems
Minoxidil	Erectile problems
Naproxen (Naprosyn)	Impotence; no ejaculation
Nicotine	Erectile problems
Nortriptyline (Aventyl, Pamelor)	Impotence
Perphenazine (Trilafon)	Decreased or no ejaculation
Phenelzine (Nardil)	Impotence; retarded or no ejaculation; difficulty achieving orgasm (men and women)
Phenoxybenzamine (Dibenzyline)	No ejaculation
Phenytoin (Dilantin and others)	Decreased sexual activity
Pindolol (Visken)	Impotence
Prazosim (Minipress)	Impotence; priapism
Progesterone (Provera)	Decreased desire; impotence
Propantheline bromide (Pro-Banthine and others)	Impotence
Propranolol (Inderal)	Loss of desire (men and women); impotence
Protriptyline (Vivactil)	Loss of desire; impotence
Ranitidine (Zantac)	Loss of desire; impotence
Reserpine	Decreased desire; impotence; decreased or no ejaculation

Drug	**Adverse Effect**
Spironolactone (Aldactone)	Decreased desire; impotence
Steroids (Cortisone, Prednisone)	Decreased desire; impotence
Thiazide diuretics (Hygroton, hydrochloro-thiazide, and others)	Impotence
Thioridazine (Mellaril)	Impotence; priapism; delayed, decreased, painful, retrograde, or no ejaculation
Thiothixene (Navane)	Spontaneous ejaculations
Timolol (Blocadren; Timolide)	Decreased desire; impotence
Tranylcypromine (Parnate)	Impotence; spontaneous erections
Trazodone (Desyrel)	Priapism; increased desire (women); retrograde ejaculation
Trifluoperazine (Stelazine)	Decreased, painful, or no ejaculation; spontaneous ejaculations

Index